IMMUNOSCINTIGRAPHY
Practical Aspects and Clinical Applications

IMMUNOSCINTIGRAPHY
Practical Aspects and Clinical Applications

A. C. PERKINS

Department of Medical Physics
University Hospital
Queen's Medical Centre
Nottingham,
United Kingdom

M. V. PIMM

Cancer Research Campaign Laboratories
University of Nottingham
Nottingham,
United Kingdom

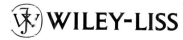 WILEY-LISS

A JOHN WILEY & SONS, INC., PUBLICATION
New York • Chichester • Brisbane • Toronto • Singapore

While the authors, editors, and publisher believe that drug selection and dosage and the specifications and usage of equipment and devices, as set forth in this book, are in accord with current recommendations and practice at the time of publication, they accept no legal responsibility for any errors or omissions, and make no warranty, express or implied, with respect to material contained herein. In view of ongoing research, equipment modifications, changes in governmental regulations and the constant flow of information relating to drug therapy, drug reactions and the use of equipment and devices, the reader is urged to review and evaluate the information provided in the package insert or instructions for each drug, piece of equipment or device for, among other things, any changes in the instructions or indications of dosage or usage and for added warnings and precautions.

Recognizing the importance of preserving what has been written, it is a policy of John Wiley & Sons, Inc. to have books of enduring value published in the United States printed on acid-free paper, and we exert our best efforts to that end.

Library of Congress Cataloging-in-Publication Data

Perkins, A.C.
    Immunoscintigraphy: practical aspects and clinical applications/
by A.C. Perkins and M.V. Pimm.
        p.   cm.
    Includes bibliographical references and index.
    ISBN 0-471-56072-3
    1. Radioimmunoimaging. I. Pimm, M.V. II. Title.
    [DNLM: 1. Antibodies, Monoclonal—diagnostic use. 2. Antibodies,
Monoclonal—isolation & purification. 3. Isotope Labeling—methods.
4. Neoplasms—radionuclide imaging. QZ 241 P448i]
RC78.7.R38P47   1991
616.07′57—dc20
DNLM/DLC
for Library of Congress   90-13155
                                                                CIP

Contents

Preface

The use of radiolabelled antibodies in clinical diagnosis has had a slow evolution. Starting with a concept that originated at the beginning of the century, it has taken the fusion of previously unrelated scientific specialities to result in a technique that is only now capable of providing diagnostic information relevant to a broad range of clinical specialities. Much of the technology involved in the production of radiolabelled antibodies suitable for clinical administration is poorly understood by the majority of clinical and paramedical staff within hospital departments. This book is primarily intended to be a handbook of immunoscintigraphy aimed at nuclear medicine personnel such as nuclear medicine physicians, radiologists, medical physicists, radiopharmacists, technicians, and radiographers, who are now beginning to use antibodies for routine clinical investigations. It should also be of interest to workers in research laboratories and the radiopharmaceutical industry. We have not set out to review the entire scope of immunoscintigraphy but have emphasised the practical aspects of this rapidly developing field so as to provide a basis for the future developments that are now inevitable.

Acknowledgments

This book has arisen from ten years' practical experience of imaging with radiolabelled monoclonal antibodies. The authors would like to thank their friends and families for support with this work. In particular we would like to thank our colleagues in the departments of Cancer Research, Medical Physics, Radiology, Surgery, Obstetrics and Gynaecology, and Radiotherapy at University Hospital, Nottingham.

Commonly Used Abbreviations and Terms

Ab: Antibody
AFP: Alpha fetoprotein
APF: Activated platelet factor
Ag: Antigen
Bq: Bequerel
CEA: Carcinoembryonic antigen
Ci: Curie
CT: Computed tomography
Da: Dalton
DTPA: Diethylene triamine pentaacetic acid
DTPAA: Diethylene triamine penta-acetic acid anhydride
EDTA: Ethylenediaminetetraacetic acid
ELISA: Enzyme-linked immunosorbent assay
EMA: Epithelial membrane antigen
Fab: Antigen-binding fragment (of antibody)
F(ab')$_2$:   Bivalent antigen-binding fragment
FACS: Fluorescent activated cell sorter
Fc: Crystallisable fragment (of antibody)
Fg: Fragment
FDA: Food and Drug Administration
GP: Glycoprotein
HAHA: Human anti-human antibody
HAMA: Human anti-mouse antibody
HCG: Human chorionic gonadotrophin

HIG: Human immunoglobulin
HMFG: Human milk fat globule
HMW: High molecular weight
HMWA: High-molecular-weight antigen
HPLC: High-performance liquid chromatography
HSA: Human serum albumin
IC: Immune complex
Ig: Immunoglobulin
IgG: Gamma immunoglobulin
IgM: Macro immunoglobulin
IS: Immunoscintigraphy
LSqCC: Lung squamous cell carcinoma
MAA: Melanoma-associated antigen
MAB: Monoclonal antibody
MBq: Mega bequerel
MOAB: Monoclonal antibody
NCA: Normal cross-reacting antigen
NF: Normalisation factor
NSLC: Non small-cell lung carcinoma
OD: Optical density
PBS: Phosphate-buffered saline
PLAP: Placental alkaline phosphatase
RAID: Radioimmunodetection
RCP: Radiochemical purity
RES: Reticuloendothelial system
RIA: Radioimmunoassay
RIS: Radioimmunoscintigraphy
RIT: Radioimmunotherapy

ROI: Region of interest   SqCC: Squamous cell carcinoma
SCLC: Small-cell lung carcinoma   TAA: Tumour-associated antigen
SDS-PAGE: Sodium dodecyl sulphate   TAG: Tumour-associated
              polyacrylamide gel   glycoprotein
              electrophoresis   TLC: Thin layer chromatography
SPECT: Single photon emission   TRIS: Tris (hydroxymethyl)
              computed tomography   aminomethane

1 Production, Purification, and Quality Control of Antibodies for Immunoscintigraphy

ANTIBODIES

Antibodies, or immunoglobulins, are produced by the body in response to the presence of foreign materials (antigens). Antibodies possess specific binding regions which recognise the corresponding site or *determinant* on the antigen. Antibodies combine physically, rather than chemically, with the specific antigen against which they were induced. In certain cases this combination of antibody and antigen initiates a series of biological processes which result in destruction and elimination of the antigen.

An antigen can have several different determinants (epitopes) each of which can stimulate the production of a different antibody. This stimulation involves the activation of a class of lymphocytes called B lymphocytes. Each B lymphocyte has the ability to differentiate into a plasma cell which then secretes antibody. Each B lymphocyte produces a single type of plasma cell which produces a specific antibody against a single antigenic determinant. Thus if animals are immunised with an antigen, they produce and secrete into their blood a mixture of antibodies each against a different determinant on the antigen. These antibodies are derived from many different stimulated B lymphocytes and are a heterogeneous mixture of many different types of antibody. Because they are the product of many different individual populations, or clones, of B lymphocytes, they are referred to as polyclonal antibodies. Monoclonal antibodies are produced using cell culture techniques. These are homogeneous in nature being secreted by a clone from a single cell line.

Antibody Structure

Immunoglobulins (Igs) are proteins. There are five main classes of immunoglobulin, IgG, IgM, IgA, IgE, and IgD. Each class of antibody serves a different function of immunity and defence. The commonest immunoglobulins are IgG and IgM, and these are the types most frequently produced as a result of the monoclonal antibody procedure (see below).

The IgG antibodies are made up of two long and two short amino acid chains referred to as *heavy* (H) and *light* (L) chains.

1

Heavy chains have molecular weights of about 50,000 daltons and light chains of about 25,000, so the whole IgG molecule has a molecular weight of about 150,000 daltons. In mice there are four types of heavy chain. Both heavy (gamma) chains in each molecule are the same, and so there are four different types, or isotypes, of IgG, referred to as IgG1, IgG2a, IgG2b, and IgG3. The first three are the commonest type of immunoglobulin naturally produced by mice and therefore the commonest IgG isotypes produced as murine monoclonal antibodies. There are two types of light chain, referred to as *kappa* and *lambda*. Again each immunoglobulin's light chains are of the same type. The kappa is the predominant type and consequently the most frequently encountered in monoclonal antibodies.

The four chains of the immunoglobulin molecule are held together by disulphide bonds. Both heavy and light chains are folded into three or four loop and sheet-like structures termed domains. Thus the three-dimensional structure of the molecule is quite complex, but it is usual to depict the structure schematically as a Y shape shown in Figure 1.1. The combining site of the antibody, that is the part which recognises the antigen, is at the end of the molecule which has both light and heavy chains. This is the variable region of the immunoglobulin molecule, where variations in amino acid sequences occur in both the heavy and light chains and confer upon each antibody its unique antigen-binding properties. The combining site is formed by a combination of the terminal parts of both the heavy and light chains. Since there are two such structures in each IgG molecule, each has two combining sites, a property referred to as bivalency.

The basic structure of the IgM immunoglobulins is similar to that of IgG, with either kappa or lambda light chains and one

sort of heavy chain (mu chains). Here, however, the molecule is formed essentially of five IgG-like subunits held together by another protein chain (the J chain), so that its overall molecular weight is about 900,000, and it has ten antigen-combining sites potentially available to react with antigen, although in practice, because of the size and shape of the molecule, each site may not be able to come into contact with the antigen.

Antibodies bind physically to the antigens which induced their formation. This interaction is essentially an ionic, non-covalent interaction, and is in fact an equilibrium between bound and free antibody and antigen. The Law of Mass Action applies to this interaction and the equilibrium constant, K from the following classic equation:

$$K = \frac{[AbAg]}{[Ab][Ag]}$$

is a measure of the strength of antibody–antigen interaction. This affinity, or more correctly the avidity of a monoclonal antibody, is expressed in units of litres/mol. Most antibodies have K values in the range 10^6–10^9 l/mol, but some have values up to 10^{12} l/mol. Generally it can be expected that the higher the K values, the better the binding of antibody will be to its target antigen.

Monoclonal Antibody Production

Throughout this century attempts have been made to identify specific antigens in human pathological lesions, especially tumours, which could be the targets for antibody therapy. The early attempts were carried out by immunisation of animals with human tissues (mainly tumour cells). These procedures may have produced antibodies with some degree of specificity for

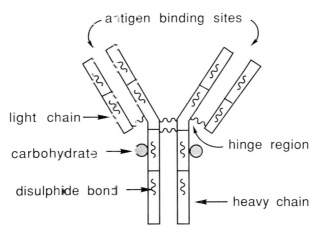

Fig. 1.1. Schematic representation of the structure of an IgG antibody molecule. It consists essentially of four protein chains, linked together by disulphide bonds. There are two heavy (H) and two light (L) chains. There are two sites which recognise antigen and these involve sites at the ends of both the heavy and light chains.

the lesion, but there was simultaneous production of other antibodies against a multitude of other normal tissue antigens so that the resulting antiserum (comprising polyclonal antibodies) would react with many normal tissues. Although it is possible to separate specific antibodies from such mixtures by the use of immunoabsorbents, this requires the availability of the target antigen in pure form. Such purified antigens were generally not available, and often the very objective of this sort of immunisation was to see whether such antigens even existed.

Theoretically, if single lymphocytes or plasma cells could be separated from animals producing polyclonal antiserum and grown in isolation, each of these clones would be producing a single species of antibody, or monoclonal antibody. These antibodies could be tested for specific reaction only against the target lesion and could be available for in vivo investigation. The fundamental problem in this case is that such antibody-producing cells cannot be maintained in vitro. The breakthrough in this area came in the 1970s when Kohler and Milstein (1975) recog-

nised that malignant forms of antibody-producing cells, myeloma cells, can survive virtually indefinitely in in vitro culture and can continue to produce immunoglobulin. They showed that using recombinant genetics it was possible to hybridise such a myeloma cell with a B lymphocyte to construct hybrid cells (hybridomas) which secrete antibody determined by the B lymphocyte and which are virtually immortal due to the malignant nature of the myeloma.

The now standard hybridoma technology is to immunise an animal, usually a mouse (but sometimes a rat) with the antigen or target tissue such as tumour cells, and to fuse lymphocytes prepared from its spleen (rich in B lymphocytes) with a specially selected and cultured myeloma line from the same strain of animal (Fig. 1.2.). The myeloma lines used are those that do not normally secrete their own immunoglobulin, so that only the antibody dictated by the lymphocytes will be secreted. There are a number of techniques for encouraging cells to fuse together, but fusion is most usually induced by the presence of polyethylene glycol in the tissue culture medium.

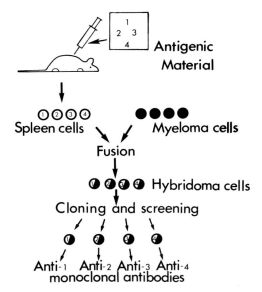

Fig. 1.2. Production of a monoclonal antibody. Animals, usually mice, are immunised with the antigenic material. Lymphocytes, generally taken from the spleen, are fused with myeloma cells to give hybridoma cells. These are then cloned to give a number of hybridomas. Each of the hybridomas generated will be producing monoclonal antibody against a different antigen present within the original immunising material or against different determinants on the same antigen. The clones therefore need screening for production of antibody against the particular antigen of interest.

Following fusion, unfused B lymphocytes are not able to survive in culture and die out. The cell population would therefore consist of the progeny of the hybrid cells, producing antibodies, and the progeny of any unfused myeloma cells. To prevent the cell population becoming overgrown with myeloma cells, an added step in the handling of the fused cells is to add a mixture of hypoxanthine, aminopterin, and thymidine (HAT) to the culture medium, which is toxic to the myeloma cells but not to hybrid cells (where resistance to this mixture is conferred by metabolic characteristics derived from the spleen cell). Thus the only cells which can survive continued culture are the hybrid cells.

Following fusion and selection, the mass cultures consist of a mixture of different hybridoma types producing antibodies against different antigens or different epitopes of the same antigen. The culture medium from these mass cultures can be tested at this stage to find out whether antibodies reactive with the antigen or specifically with the tissue of interest are being produced. The next part of the process towards monoclonal antibody production is to clone the hybridoma cells. This is done usually by a process of limiting dilution in which cell suspensions are diluted so much that the small volume which is to be inoculated into wells of microculture plates will contain on average only one cell. Following incubation, the wells containing growth are selected and their medium tested for antibody against the antigen. Cells from positive wells are grown up further, and usually cloned at least one more time before they are regarded as monoclonal and their antibodies as monoclonal antibodies.

One of the great advantages of this technology is that as well as generating monoclonal antibodies against known antigens, it can also be used to search for other as yet unidentified antigens. For example, if mice were originally immunised with tumour tissues, clones can be tested for production of antibody reactive with that type of tumour (for example, colon carcinoma) but not with the corresponding normal tissue (for example, normal colonic tissue). Many of the human tumour-associated antigens which are of interest for tumour imaging and in the understanding of tumour structural biochemistry have been identified in this way (Reisfeld and Cheresh, 1987). Thus monoclonal antibodies are useful not only in immunoscintigraphy directed against specific antigens, but also in their isolation and characterisation. This ability to isolate the antigen identified by the monoclonal antibody means that purified antigen can then be used to immunise animals to generate further antibodies against the same antigen. These "second generation" antibodies may have potential advantages over the original antibody in a number of ways, such as different avidity or different isotypes with better fragmentation characteristics (see below).

Although these monoclonal antibody-defined antigens associated with tumours are antigens in the sense that they are identified by antibodies, it should be recognised that they are most likely not antigenic in patients and that patients are not producing any immune response to them. To call them simply *tumour antigens* is a misnomer which can lead to some confusion.

Hybridoma technology as outlined above is now a fairly routine technique in immunology, but is nevertheless a lengthy procedure. Animals which are to provide spleen cells for fusions are generally immunised several times with antigenic material, over a period of several weeks or months. Subsequent fusion, screening, cloning, recloning, and testing of hybridomas takes many more weeks. Once cloned and established, hybridomas can be cultured in conventional tissue culture systems. Theoretically, hybridoma cells will grow indefinitely and continue to produce monoclonal antibody. In practice it is sometimes found that clones are unstable and will start to produce only low levels of antibody or sometimes stop antibody production altogether. Thus it is important to preserve seed lots of each hybridoma as soon as it has been established as monoclonal and shown to be producing antibody of interest. These seed lots can be used periodically to initiate new cultures of the hybridoma.

Hybridomas secreting monoclonal antibodies can be grown *in vitro* in tissue culture, and the spent medium from the cultures used for purification of the antibody. Large scale *in vitro* culture is expensive because of the cost of the medium and particularly because of the cost of serum, usually foetal calf serum, which is essential for cell growth and has to be used as a medium supplement. Recently, suitable non-serum protein supplements have been introduced, and this means that large-scale growth of hybridomas is becoming cheaper. Hybridomas can be grown in static flask culture, in roller bottles or, as is now becoming more common, in suspension culture in long-term, fermenter-type culture vessels with continual input of fresh medium and tap-off of antibody-rich medium.

At one time an alternative to *in vitro* growth was to grow the hybridoma cells *in vivo*. Generally the original myeloma cell line used for the fusion is from the same strain of mice which is immunised with the antigen to provide spleen cells. Thus the resulting hybridoma can grow in that strain of mice, with the growth potential coming from the malignant nature of the myeloma. The usual way to grow the hybridoma is as an ascites by injecting hybridoma cells intraperitoneally. Mice would eventually have to be killed as they became moribund with the load of ascites tumour. Ascitic fluid and serum from these mice are rich in monoclonal antibody which has continued to be secreted by the hybridoma. This *in vivo* method to produce ascites grown antibody was widely used in early work to produce antibody for immunoscintigraphy but has now generally been superseded by *in vitro* culture. The *in vivo* method has the disadvantages that prolonged *in vivo* exposure of the antibody can lead to some loss of antigen-binding activity, purified antibody can be contaminated with normal immunoglobulins from the mouse, and viral and other microbial contamination of the purified antibody is more likely from mice than it is from sterile *in vitro* techniques.

Human monoclonal antibodies. Most monoclonal antibodies currently available for immunoscintigraphy are of murine (i.e., mouse or rat origin). As discussed in Chapter 6, this volume, there are problems associated with the clinical use of such monoclonal antibodies, essentially due to the fact that they are foreign proteins and as such can evoke adverse immunological reaction in patients. An alternative to murine antibodies would be to produce human monoclonal antibodies. However, this requires the production of an immune response to antigens associated with the target lesion in patients so that their lymphocytes can be fused with an appropriate human myeloma. With some antigens of interest this might not be possible; for example, it is doubtful whether humans would produce an immune response against, say, their own platelets to provide hybridomas producing antibodies for imaging of thrombi. It is with tumours that this approach has attracted most attention so far, since it is thought possible (although by no means certain) that patients may perhaps be responding to new antigens associated only with the tumour cells. Thus lymphocytes, either from peripheral blood or in some cases isolated from lymph nodes draining tumour sites, have been fused with human myeloma or lymphoblastoid cells. Although there are now some reports of the generation of monoclonal antibodies against tumour-associated antigens (Kjeldsen et al., 1988), very often this procedure produces hybridomas secreting antibodies cross-reactive with normal tissues, and has probably selected patients' auto-antibodies against normal tissues. Furthermore, these are often IgM antibodies against intracellular rather than cell surface antigens, and the hybridomas are often not stable.

Chimeric antibodies. An alternative method of producing human monoclonal antibodies, theoretically applicable to any antigen of interest against which murine monoclonal antibodies can be generated, is to use genetic engineering to produce chimeric antibodies (Olsson, 1985; Reichmann et al., 1988; Brown et al., 1987). Here murine genes coding just for the hypervariable regions of the heavy and light chains are introduced into a cell together with human genes coding for the rest of the immunoglobulin molecule. The antibodies produced by these hybridomas contain partly human immunoglobulin protein and partly murine immunoglobulin protein, and can be constructed so that the majority of the molecule is human and only a minor component, the antigen-combining (hypervariable) region, is murine. Although not yet in wide clinical use, these chimeric antibodies could potentially overcome some of the problems associated with adverse reactions to the murine immunoglobulin.

Monoclonal Antibody Purification

Tissue culture supernatants of *in vitro* grown hybridomas contain usually a few tens of micrograms of monoclonal antibody/millilitre of fluid. There are a number of immunochemical ways to purify this antibody, but the most widely used with IgG antibodies has been to exploit the property of a staphylococcal protein, Protein A, to bind non-specifically to immunoglobulins. Protein A immobilised onto an inert support is widely available commercially, and can be packed into chromatography columns. Cells are removed from tissue culture medium by centrifugation or filtration, and the medium is then pumped through the Protein A column, which adsorbs immunoglobulin. The column of Protein A can then be washed to remove unbound materials and the adsorbed antibody eluted off, usually by reducing the pH from the approximately neutral values of the culture medium to pH 2 or pH 3. Different immunoglobulin isotypes bind with different efficiencies to Protein A, this being pH-dependent. Those of the

IgG1 isotype bind most poorly at neutral pH, but binding as part of the purification procedure can usually be achieved satisfactorily by raising the pH of the supernatant to pH 8 before application to the Protein A.

An alternative non-specific adsorbent for immunoglobulins which can be used to purify monoclonal antibodies is hydroxylapatite. Like Protein A, this binds immunoglobulins, but bound material can then be eluted, in this case by increasing the salt concentration in the buffer used to wash through the column.

Similar procedures can be used to purify ascites grown monoclonal antibody, but here it has to be borne in mind that any normal mouse immunoglobulin present in the ascites fluid will usually be co-purified with the monoclonal antibody. This can be overcome to some extent by eluting bound immunoglobulin at the pH or salt concentration appropriate for the particular isotype of the monoclonal antibody, thus excluding any other isotypes of normal immunoglobulin.

IgM antibodies do not bind to Protein A, but a number of alternative methods are available for their purification. For example, IgM antibodies are particularly rich in carbohydrate, and this causes them to bind to some plant lectins. Affinity chromatography with immobilised lentil lectin (which is commercially available in this form) is carried out by running IgM containing supernatants through a column of the material and then eluting the bound antibody, usually by the application of excess sugar such as methyl-mannoside. The high molecular weight of IgM, higher than other materials likely to be present in hybridoma culture supernatants, can also be exploited, and antibody can sometimes be isolated simply by gel filtration on appropriate media.

Monoclonal antibodies purified in these ways are then usually returned to isotonic saline solutions, usually buffered at pH 7, and stored either by refrigeration (although they will require sterilisation, usually by membrane filtration) or frozen at −20°C or at lower temperatures. However, it is imperative to establish that the purified antibody has retained its immunological activity by testing with antigen in appropriate assays.

Antibody Fragments

Treatment of immunoglobulins with proteolytic enzymes was used by early workers for the determination of antibody structure and is now a routine procedure to prepare fragments of monoclonal antibodies with different properties. These antibody fragments have quite different biodistribution characteristics from intact antibody, and this has been exploited in immunoscintigraphy in an attempt to increase target to non-target ratios.

$F(ab')_2$ fragments. One widely used enzyme, pepsin, acts adjacent to the disulphide bonds which hold the two heavy chains together. This cleaves off the tail end of the molecule and leaves a fragment of about 100,000 daltons which still has the bivalent antigen-binding part and which is termed the $F(ab')_2$ fragment (F for fragment, ab_2 for antibody binding in bivalent form) (Fig. 1.3).

Fab fragments. The other widely used enzyme, papain, removes a larger part of the heavy chains, still linked by disulphide bonds to give a fragment termed the Fc (F for fragment, and c for crystallisable, since early on it was found that such fragments could be crystallised) and two identical fragments each of 50,000 daltons, each with a single antibody-binding site and termed Fab fragments (Fig. 1.3).

This is rather a simplified view of monoclonal antibody fragmentation, and in practice not all antibodies respond so favourably (Parham, 1986). For example, the different isotypes require different

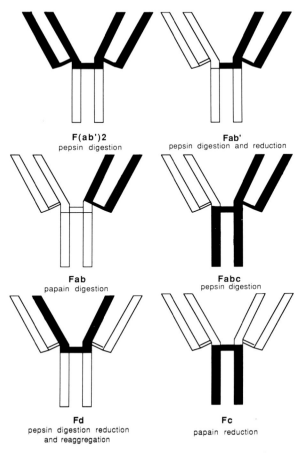

Fig. 1.3. Antibody molecules can be broken down by enzymes into fragments. Pepsin removes part of the Fc region of the antibody to give a F(ab')₂ fragment which still has two combining sites but a lower molecular weight (about 100,000 daltons) than intact antibody. Papain breaks the molecule into smaller Fab fragments, which have only one combining site and a lower molecular weight (about 50,000 daltons) and Fc fragments which have no antigen combining sites. Enzymatic treatment of antibody for the production of Fab', Fabc, Fd, and Fc is also shown.

concentrations and times of incubation with pepsin to yield F(ab')₂ fragments. Pepsin digestion can also be used with some isotypes to produce Fab fragments. These are very slightly different from those made with papain, and are designated Fab'. From one of the isotypes, IgG2b, it is virtually impossible to produce F(ab')₂ fragments, pepsin digestion producing Fab' fragments and a fragment with only one Fab combining site and an intact Fc portion (this fragment being termed the Fab/c fragment).

The different isotypes also respond differently to papain, requiring different conditions of incubation and sometimes the addition of cysteine to produce Fab fragments. It should be borne in mind that in the fragmentation of monoclonal antibodies (because each is, by definition, unique), procedures suitable for the fragmentation of one antibody may not be suitable for another, even of the same isotype. Pilot studies are required with each antibody to optimise the enzyme treatment conditions.

The most commonly used fragments of monoclonal antibodies in immunoscintigraphy are the $F(ab')_2$ and Fab. Other fragments can be made, using other enzymes, but their properties in relation to immunoscintigraphy have not yet been explored. Of particular interest could be the univalent Fab/c fragments and the bivalent Facb fragments.

Fragments of monoclonal antibodies can be purified from enzyme digests using procedures similar to those used in the original isolation of the antibody from culture supernatant. For example, Protein A can be used to remove any remaining intact antibody (by binding to the Fc portion) or free Fc fragments. $F(ab')_2$ and Fab fragments, being of quite different molecular weights, can usually be separated by gel filtration chromatography.

Bispecific Antibodies

Most immunoscintigraphy studies reported so far have been with monoclonal antibodies radiolabelled with the appropriate radionuclide. An alternative approach is to administer antibody without a radiolabel to pre-target to the lesion, and then to administer a radiolabelled tracer capable of localising onto the antibody in the lesion.

One possibility for such pre-targeted immunoscintigraphy is to use a bispecific antibody, sometimes called a bifunctional antibody. This is an antibody in which one of the combining sites can react with the antigen in the target tissue and the other combining site with an appropriate radiolabelled tracer. These are sometimes called hybrid antibodies, being a cross between two antibodies, each with different specificities. For example, there are recent reports of the use of such bispecific antibodies in imaging of tumours. In one study (Stickney et al., 1989) one combining site of the antibody reacted with a tumour-associated antigen (CEA), and the other combining site with an EDTA derivative of bleomycin, which could be labelled with In-111.

These bispecific antibodies can be produced chemically by dissociating each antibody in a purified form to its Fab fragment and then chemically cross-linking them to form $F(ab)_2$-like molecules. The bispecific antibody can be purified from any remaining Fab fragments by gel filtration chromatography. Alternatively two hybridomas can be fused together, in the same way that each was originally generated by fusion of a myeloma and a lymphocyte. The resultant hybrid hybridoma is sometimes referred to as a quadroma, as it is the product of the fusion of four cell types. These quadromas produce three different types of monoclonal antibody, these being the antibodies from each of the parent hybridomas and a hybrid between the two. Purification of the hybrid from the other antibodies can be difficult, and is technically most easy with immunoabsorbants of the two separate antigens, if these are available in purified form.

Target Antigens of Interest for Immunoscintigraphy

Monoclonal antibodies for immunoscintigraphy have been produced against a number of different target lesions (Table 1.1). These include antibodies to fibrin and platelets for thrombus imaging, granulocytes for imaging abscess and sites of inflammation, myosin for myocardial infarction, bacteria for localized infection, and tumour antigens for the detection particularly of recurrent or metastatic disease.

If the monoclonal antibody is not sufficiently specific for the target lesion, this will affect image quality. Any reaction of the antibody against normal tissues expressing the antigen could possibly lead, via immunological mechanisms, to some

TABLE 1.1. Target Antigens of Interest
for Immunoscintigraphy

Antigen associated with	Potential for imaging
Tumours	Primary, recurrent and metastatic cancer
Fibrin	Thrombi, tumours
Platelets	Thrombi
Myosin	Myocardial infarction, Tumours
Granulocytes	Inflammatory lesions
Bacteria	Localised infection
Parasites	Parasitic infection

damage of that tissue. With all monoclonal antibodies it is desirable that only the target lesion will produce the defined antigen. This is certainly the hope with antibodies to tumour antigens. The monoclonal antibody should be shown to be reactive with tumour tissue by, for example, immunohistology. This method can also be used to assess the cross-reactivity of the monoclonal antibody against normal human tissues. Extensive cross-reactivity, or even limited cross-reactivity against some tissues, should preclude the clinical use of the antibody.

In some cases the monoclonal antibody cannot really be target-specific, for example, with anti-platelet antibodies for thrombus imaging and anti-granulocyte antibodies for imaging sites of inflammation. In these circumstances the monoclonal antibody reacts with the cells in the circulation, and it is only after their accumulation at the pathological site that imaging of the lesion is possible. Even here, though, the antibodies should be screened for reaction against other normal tissues prior to use.

In the case of monoclonal antibodies to fibrin, used for imaging thrombi, it is possible to produce antibodies reacting with fibrin, such as is present in thrombi, and not with circulating fibrinogen (Knight et al., 1988). With anti-myosin antibodies for imaging myocardial infarction, the antibodies are reacting with normal myosin, but their ability to image these lesions depends on antigen being available for antibody recognition because of the damage to myocardial cell membranes at the site of the lesion.

Interestingly, the cross-reaction of some monoclonal antibodies can be usefully exploited. For example, some antibodies against CEA, and its normally occurring counterpart NCA, react with the same sort of antigen expressed on granulocytes and have been used for imaging inflammatory lesions (Seybold et al., 1988). Anti-myosin monoclonal antibody, intended for imaging of myocardial infarction, has been successfully used to image rhabdomyosarcomas and leiomyosarcomas (Cox et al., 1988).

One of the clinically most widely evaluated type of lesion so far has been cancer. The aim here is to generate antibodies reactive with abnormal antigens which are associated with tumour tissue but which are not present in normal tissues. Monoclonal antibodies have been produced showing reactivity against a variety of human cancers, including carcinomas of colon, rectum, breast, ovary, bladder, and pancreas, as well as bone and soft tissue sarcomas, melanoma, and leukaemias. The majority of these are mouse monoclonal antibodies; a few are of rat origin. Often several different antibodies are available against any one type of malignancy.

As part of their selection and production, antibodies against tumour-associated antigens will have been tested for reactivity against malignant rather than corresponding normal tissues. However, they are probably not reacting with truly tumour-specific antigens, but only with antigens which are preferentially or inappropriately expressed in malignancy. One class of such antigens is the oncofoetal cell antigens. These are expressed in some malignant and foetal cells, but either absent from or expressed in lower levels in normal adult tissues. Carcinoembryonic antigen (CEA) is the most widely examined in the context of immunoscintigraphy. This is a complex material, with both protein and carbohydrate determinants, and is widely associated particularly with colorectal cancers. Another such antigen is alpha-foetoprotein (AFP), produced particularly in hepatocellular carcinoma and teratoblastomas of testis and ovary. These types of antigens have the advantage that their structure is relatively well known, and they are available in purified form, aiding considerably in immunisation of animals and in the screening of hybridoma products. Other antigens of interest are placental alkaline phosphatase, in ovarian tumours and epidermal growth factor receptor.

The nature and function of many other monoclonal antibody-defined tumour-associated antigens are relatively unknown, and their original description has often been by way of the production of monoclonal antibodies against them. Elucidation of their nature is a major endeavour in itself (Reisfeld and Cheresh, 1987), but many are glycoproteins and glycolipids associated with the surface of malignant cells, either in a membrane associated form and/or secreted at the cell surface. Antibodies against antigens expressed only intracellularly are likely to be of little value in immunoscintigraphy, since antigen will not be presented to antibody in the circulation or extravascular fluid of tumours. There are one or two reported exceptions to this, but these are probably due to tissue necrosis causing local leakage of intracellular antigen.

Quality Control of Monoclonal Antibodies Intended for Human Use

Monoclonal antibody preparations intended for human use should obviously undergo preclinical toxicity testing to ensure their safety. Legislation governing such clinical development and use of new radiopharmaceuticals will differ throughout the world, and no precise rules can be given here. Investigators wishing to develop their own monoclonal antibodies for immunoscintigraphy will have to satisfy whatever legislation is in force in their own country, both with respect to the clinical administration of monoclonal antibodies and to the administration of radioactive materials. Pharmaceutical companies providing monoclonal antibodies for clinical trials, or marketing such antibodies, will also have to satisfy current legislation. Generally the requirements of licensing bodies with regard to physicians carrying out a limited trial of antibody imaging in their own patients are less demanding than those required of a pharmaceutical company seeking a clinical trial licence or a product licence.

The very minimum quality control which the early published papers reported in pilot studies was purely for the assessment of the imaging ability of new antibodies. This generally ensured that the preparation of antibody was free of aggregates, passed pyrogenicity tests, and was sterile, as least as far as passing standard bacteriological sterility testing. But the expansion of immunoscintigraphy, from individual research centres investigating the usefulness of particular antibodies, to fuller trials which are now the interest of radiopharmaceutical companies developing antibodies for clinical trials and eventual marketing, has prompted the involvement of a number of official bodies. There are some published guidelines for the production and quality control testing of monoclonal antibodies. These include the following:

In the USA "Points to Consider in the Manufacture and Testing of Monoclonal Antibody Products for Human Use," produced by the Office of Biologics Research and Review, Center for Drugs and Biologics of the Food and Drugs Administration.

In Europe "Guidelines on the Production and Quality Control of Monoclonal Antibodies of Murine Origin Intended for Use in Man," produced by the Committee for Proprietary Medicinal Products of the Commission of the European Communities as notes to applicants for marketing authorizations (Guidelines, 1988).

In the UK "An Operation Manual for Control of Production, Preclinical Toxicology and Phase I Trials of Anti-Tumour Antibodies and Drug Antibody Conjugates," produced by a Joint Committee of The National Institute for Biological Standards and Control and The Cancer Research Campaign (Operation Manual, 1986).

It would not be appropriate to discuss in depth these documents here because they are at the stage of recommendations rather than specific legislation, the regulations will vary from country to country, and those covering manufacturers will differ from those for individual investigators. Nevertheless, certain areas common to all of these documents will be outlined here since they deal with basic matters of which anyone considering monoclonal antibody for clinical use should be aware (Table 1.2).

Seed lots of hybridomas. It is essential that multiple samples of hybridoma are

TABLE 1.2. Points to Consider in Development of a Monoclonal Antibody for Clinical Imaging Trials

1. The specificity of the monoclonal antibody for the proposed target lesion.
2. The possible production by the hybridoma culture which produces the monoclonal antibody of nucleic acids, viruses, or other microorganisms which might contaminate the final purified antibody.
3. The stability of the hybridoma in its continued production of homogeneous antibody.
4. The toxicity of the antibody itself.
5. The freedom of the purified antibody from pyrogens, viruses, and other microorganisms co-purified with the monoclonal antibody or introduced during the purification procedure.
6. The freedom of the purified and radiolabelled antibody from aggregated or damaged antibody, free radionuclide, or chemical contaminants introduced in, or arising from, the labelling procedure.

stored at an early stage in its development as seed lots for further production. These seed lots, and the monoclonal antibody produced from their culture, are definitive samples against which to compare further samples of the hybridoma and its antibody after growth *in vitro* and *in vivo*. Hybridomas can change their characteristics and it is essential to have such definitive samples so that periodically new cultures can be initiated from them, rather than simply passaging the hybridoma cells continually in tissue culture or *in vivo*. It is recommended that these seed lots should be shown to be free of bacterial, fungal, and mycoplasma contamination, and this can be assessed by conventional sterility testing procedures. The seed lots should also be shown to be free of viral contamination, although this is technically more difficult.

The minimum virus testing suggested in one of the published recommendations (Operation Manual, 1986) is to demonstrate that there is no toxicity in animals, such as suckling mice and guinea pigs, following inoculation of disrupted hybridoma cells. The ability of disrupted hybridoma to cause cytopathic effects when inoculated into cultured human or primate cells was also suggested. Other guidelines suggest a more rigorous screen for viruses, both for those which are potential contaminants and which are known to be able to infect man, and for others which, although there is no evidence for infection in man, could be a potential danger in patients already ill with other conditions, such as cancer. Such virus testing can only be performed in laboratories with experience in routine virus testing.

Culture of hybridomas. Some hybridomas are difficult to grow *in vitro,* and with those which can be grown either *in vivo* or *in vitro,* ascites growth can yield a few millilitres of fluid from each animal, containing often several milligrams of antibody, whereas *in vitro* growth to the point where the medium is exhausted (or spent) can produce usually only a few ten's of micrograms per millilitre.

In vitro culture is the preferred method of antibody production. *In vitro* growth yields antibody not subject to any *in vivo* denaturation, free of contaminating normal mouse serum immunoglobulin and free of any microorganisms from the animals. At one time *in vitro* culture invariably required supplementary tissue culture medium with animal serum, usually bovine or foetal calf serum, to enable the hybridoma cells to grow. Consideration should be given to the fact that these animal sera could potentially be contami-

nated with bovine or other viruses. Recently non-serum based protein supplements prepared from animal tissues have been introduced, partly to obviate the high cost of animal serum, but consideration obviously has to be given to possible viral contamination of these preparations too.

In many routine tissue culture situations it is common to add antibiotics to culture media, to prevent outgrowth of microorganisms if the cultures become contaminated. But it is undesirable to use in the culture of hybridomas those antibiotics (for example, penicillin or other β-lactam antibiotics) which, if they contaminated the final purified antibody, could evoke sensitivity reactions in certain individuals.

Antibody purification and quality control testing. Purification of monoclonal antibodies from ascites fluid or tissue culture medium is usually carried out by some type of affinity chromatography. The antibody is absorbed from the production materials onto, for example, Protein A, and only the adsorbed material eluted off as purified antibody. Nevertheless, it is advocated that the purification method used with any particular antibody should be shown to be capable of removing any contaminating viruses or free nucleic acids from the final product.

Once purified, it is recommended that the antibody preparation is treated to inactivate any possible contaminating viruses which have leaked through the purification. Heat treatment is one such method, and it is generally assumed that 55–60°C for a few minutes will inactivate most viruses, although there are known to be exceptions to this. Although some monoclonal antibodies are stable to this sort of treatment, others may not be, and obviously the reactivity of such heated antibody would have to be assessed.

Aggregates often form in protein solutions, and this can affect monoclonal antibodies, particularly during their physical manipulation and handling. These are likely to reduce the immunoreactivity of the preparations and increase their possible side effects in patients, particularly the immunogenicity. The standard procedure to remove these aggregates from protein solutions is to expose the solutions to high-speed centrifugation, at $100,000 \times g$ for one hour. With high-molecular-weight proteins such as antibodies this may sediment some non-aggregated protein too, and centrifugation at $50,000 \times g$, twice, is perhaps more widely used with antibodies to prevent undue loss of material.

Once purified, heat or otherwise treated and centrifuged, conventional membrane filtration of antibody solutions can be used to remove bacterial contamination almost certainly introduced during the purification procedure.

It is most practical to store antibody in aliquots suitable for labelling sufficient for a one-patient imaging dose. Thus aliquots of up to, say, one millilitre containing a few milligrams of antibody are probably most convenient. Some antibodies will be stable and retain immunological activity even for several years simply stored in standard refrigeration conditions ($4°C$), although others may require storage frozen at $-20°C$ or even lower ($-80°C$). Each antibody will require individual assessment in this respect. Frozen storage is most likely to retain the best activity of the antibody, although freeze/thawing may induce aggregate formation.

In some cases antibody will have to be modified for radiolabelling with the radionuclide required for imaging. For example, chelating groups may be covalently attached to the antibody to allow chelation of radiometals such as In-111 (see Chapter 2, this volume). It is obviously advisable to incorporate this procedure as early as possible into the preparation of the antibody after its purification.

Samples of the antibody destined for radiolabelling prior to clinical use should be tested for bacterial, fungal, and mycoplasma contamination, and some authorities would advocate virus testing also. The materials should also be tested for contamination with pyrogens, either by conventional pyrogen testing in rabbits or by the newer *in vitro* assays, if the latter are acceptable to the local regulatory authorities.

Antibody toxicity testing. It is recognised that classical toxicological studies in animals may be of only limited relevance to studies of monoclonal antibodies. Part of the problem here is that the relevant target antigen for the antibody is unlikely to be present in an animal species, so that toxicity associated with antigen–antibody interactions cannot be assessed. However, some form of toxicity testing is generally advocated, usually in two different species, for example in mice and rabbits, by the same route of injection as to be used clinically (usually intravenously). With preparations such as monoclonal antibodies, conventional lethality testing to determine an LD_{50} is inappropriate. However, the dose to be tested for adverse effects should obviously be at least as great as that to be used clinically on a dose/body weight basis, and at least ten times this dose is generally advocated. Obviously sizeable groups of animals (often 10) and the same number of control animals are needed for this. Gross pathological examination, histology on any organs found to be abnormal, and haematological examinations should be carried out following eventual sacrifice of the animals, perhaps a week or two after injection. This form of toxicity testing should identify any toxicity associated with the monoclonal antibody *per se* as a protein. It is probably sufficient to carry out this only once, on a representative batch of antibody. Each lot of the same antibody need not necessarily undergo similar testing, but would of course have to undergo sterility and pyrogen testing.

REFERENCES AND FURTHER READING

Bai, Y., Durbin, H., Hogg, N. (1984): Monoclonal antibodies specific for platelet glycoprotein react with human monocytes. Blood 64:139–146

Brown, B.A., Davis, D.L., Saltzgaber-Muller, J., Simon, P., Ho, M.K., Shaw, P.S., Stone, B.A., Sands, H., Moore, G.P. (1987): Tumor-specific genetically engineered murine/human chimeric monoclonal antibody. Cancer Res. 47:3577–3583.

Collet, B., Pellen, P., Martin, A., Moisan, A., Bourel, D., Toujas, L. (1988): Scintigraphic detection in mice of inflammatory lesions and tumours by an indium labelled monoclonal antibody directed against Mac-1 antigen. Cancer Immunol. Immunother. 26:237–242.

Cox, P.H., Verweij, J., Pillay, M., Stoter, G., Schonfeld, D. (1988): Indium-111 antimyosin for the detection of leiomyosarcoma and rhamdomyosarcoma. Eur. J. Nucl. Med. 14:50–52.

Guidelines (1988): Guidelines on the Production and Quality Control of Monoclonal Antibodies of Murine Origin Intended for Use in Man. Tibtech 6:G5–G8.

Hardy, R.R. (1986): Purification and characterisation of monoclonal antibodies. In: Weir, D.H. (ed.) Handbook of Experimental Immunology. Vol. I. Oxford: Blackwell, pp 13.1–13.3.

Khaw, B.A., Fallon, J.T., Strauss, H.W., Haber, E. (1980): Myocardial infarct imaging of antibodies to canine cardiac myosin with indium-111-diethylenetriamine pentaacetic acid. Science 209: 295–297.

Kjeldsen, T.B., Rasmussen, B.B., Rose, C., Zeuthen, J. (1988): Human-human hybridomas and human monoclonal antibodies obtained by fusion of lymph node lymphocytes from breast cancer patients. Cancer Res. 38:3208–3214.

Knight, L.C., Maurer, A.H., Ammar, I.A., Shealy, D.J., Mattis, J.A. (1988): Evaluation of indium-111-labeled anti-fibrin antibody for imaging vascular thrombi. J. Nucl. Med. 29:494–502.

Kohler, G., Milstein, C. (1975): Continuous culture of fused cells secreting antibody of predetermined specificity. Nature 256:495–497.

Locher, J.T., Seybold, K., Andres, R.Y., Schubiger, P.A., Mach, J.P., Buchegger, F. (1986): Imaging of inflammatory and infectious lesions after injection of radioiodinated monoclonal anti-granulocyte antibodies. Nucl. Med Commun. 7:689–670.

Olsson, L. (1985): Human monoclonal antibodies in cancer research. J. Natl Cancer Inst. 75:397–403.

Operation Manual (1986): An Operation Manual for Control of Production, Preclinical Toxicology, and

Phase I Trials of Anti-Tumour Antibodies and Drug Antibody Conjugates. Br. J. Cancer 54:557–568.

Parham, P. (1986): Preparation and purification of active fragments from mouse monoclonal antibodies. In: D.H. Weir (ed.): Handbook of Experimental Immunology. Vol. I. Oxford: Blackwell, pp 14.1–14.23.

Peters, A.M., Lavender, J.P., Needham, S.G., Loutifi, I., Snook, D., Epenetos, A.A., Lumley, P., Kerry, R.J., Hogg, N. (1986): Imaging thrombus with radiolabelled antibody to platelets. Br. Med. J. 293:1525–1527.

Reichmann, L., Clark, M., Waldmann, H., Winter, G. (1988): Reshaping human antibodies for therapy. Nature 332:323–327.

Reisfeld, R.A., Cheresh, D.A. (1987): Human tumour antigens. Adv. Immunol. 40:323–377.

Roseborough, S.F., Grossman, Z.D., McAfee, J.G., Kudryk, B.J., Subramanian, G., Ritter-Hrncirik, C.A., Witanowski, L.S., Tillapaugh-Fay, G., Urrutia, E., Zapf-Longo, C. (1988): Thrombus imaging with indium-111 and iodine-131-labeled fibrin specific monoclonal antibody and its F(ab')$_2$ and Fab fragments. J. Nucl. Med. 29:1212–1222.

Rubin, R.H., Young, L.S., Hansen, P., Edelman, M., Wilkinson, E., Nelles, M.J., Callahen, R., Khaw, B.A., Strauss, H.W. (1988): Specific and non-specific imaging of localized Fisher Immunotype I Pseudomonas aeruginosa infection with radiolabeled monoclonal antibody. J. Nucl. Med. 29: 651–656.

Seybold, K., Locher, J.T., Coosman, C., Andres, R.Y., Schubiger, P.A., Blauenstein, P. (1988): Immunoscintigraphic localization of inflammatory lesions: Clinical experience. Eur. J. Nucl. Med. 13: 587–593.

Som, P., Oster, Z.H., Zamora, P.O., Yamamoto, K., Sacker, D.F., Brill, A.B., Newall, K.D., Rhoses, B.A. (1986): Radioimaging of experimental thrombi in dogs using technetium-99m-labeled monoclonal antibody fragments reactive with human platelets. J. Nucl. Med. 27:1315–1320.

Stanker, L.H., Vanderlaan, M., Juarez-Salinas, H. (1985): One step purification of mouse monoclonal antibodies from ascites fluid by hydroxylapatite chromatography. J. Immunol. Methods 76: 157–169.

Stickney, D.R., Slater, J.B., Kirk, G.A., Ahlem, C., Chang, C-H, Frinke, H.M. (1989): Bifunctional antibody: ZCE/CHA Indium-111 BLEDTA-IV clinical imaging in colorectal carcinoma. Antibody, Immunoconjugates, and Radiopharmaceuticals 2: 1–13.

Stuttle, A.W.J., Peters, A.M., Loutfi, I., Lumley, P., George, P., Lavender, J.P. (1988): Use of anti-platelet monoclonal antibody F(ab')$_2$ fragment for imaging thrombus. Nucl. Med. Commun. 9:647–655.

Tom, B.H., Allison J.P. (eds.) (1983): Hybridomas and Cellular Immortality. New York: Plenum Press.

Wright, G.L. (ed.) (1984): Monoclonal Antibodies and Cancer. New York: Marcel Dekker.

2 | Preparation and Characterization of Radiolabelled Antibodies

RADIOLABELLING OF MONOCLONAL ANTIBODIES

This chapter describes how antibodies may be radiolabelled and how the characteristics of the labelled preparations may be determined. A number of radionuclides already in use in nuclear medicine have been used to label monoclonal antibodies for clinical imaging studies. All are gamma emitters since their biodistribution has to be imaged externally (Table 2.1).

There has been much work in the past with iodine-131, and although this continues to be widely used, its future use is more likely to be in therapy rather than diagnosis. This radionuclide is readily available, and cheap, and techniques for easy attachment of radioiodines to proteins such as antibodies have been available for many years. Iodine-131 has disadvantages in that its energy of gamma emission (364 keV) means that it is poorly collimated and inefficiently detected by the sodium iodide crystals in standard gamma cameras. In addition, its long physical half-life (8 days) and associated beta emission pose problems of radiation doses to patients. Another radionuclide of iodine, iodine-123, has gamma emission at 159 keV (which is more efficiently detected by modern gamma cameras), no beta emission, and can be used to label antibodies in the same way as iodine-131. Iodine-123 has a half-life of 13 hours and does have the disadvantage of high cost and poor availability. The short physical half-life of iodine-123 does mean that high activities of radiolabel might have to be given in circumstances where imaging is required more than 24 hours after administration. Although it is considered that maximal uptake of antibody occurs some 2 to 3 days following administration, acceptable imaging results may be obtained within 24 hours using the lower energy short-lived radionuclides such as iodine-123. In the case of these radionuclides, the low energy of emission and high efficiency of photon detection result in a high signal-to-noise content within the images, thereby producing good clinical results.

Following the early successful imaging, particularly of tumours, with radioiodine-labelled monoclonal antibodies, techniques were, and continue to be, developed for labelling antibodies with radiometals frequently used in nuclear medicine, i.e., indium-111 and technetium-

17

TABLE 2.1. Factors Affecting the Choice of Radionuclide for Antibody Labelling

Radionuclide	Availability	Cost	Physical half-life	Principal gamma energies (keV)
^{123}I	Poor	High	13 h	159
^{131}I	Good	Low	8 d	364
^{111}In	Good	Moderate	67 h	173
				247
^{67}Ga	Good	Moderate	78 h	185
				300
^{99m}Tc	Good	Low	6 h	141

99m. Of these, indium-111 has been the most widely used to date. Its gamma emissions at 173 and 247 keV, and physical half-life of 2.8 days, are very suitable for imaging the biodistribution of monoclonal antibodies. Technically simple methods are now available for its attachment to monoclonal antibodies. Technetium's gamma energy of 141 keV is ideally suited to gamma cameras. Technetium is cheap and readily available in most nuclear medicine departments. Its short physical half-life of only six hours, an advantage in many nuclear medicine investigations, restricts imaging to within 24 hours of administration. A number of methods for technetium-99m labelling of monoclonal antibodies have been described and are technically more complex than those for indium-111. Gallium-67 with gamma emissions at 93, 185, and 300 keV and a 3.25-day physical half-life has also been used to label monoclonal antibodies. Published labelling techniques are complex, and no simple reliable methods are available to date.

Antibody Labelling With Radioiodines

Radioiodination methods available for antibody labelling involve either direct or indirect attachment of iodine to the pro-tein. Direct attachment has so far been the most widely used for radiolabelling monoclonal antibodies for clinical use, although newer developments in indirect labelling may produce materials for clinical evaluation.

Direct labelling. In direct labelling, radioiodine, available from many suppliers as a sodium iodide solution, is treated with a mild oxidizing agent in the presence of the antibody. Cationic iodine (I+) is presumed to be formed under these oxidizing conditions, and there is an electrophilic aromatic substitution into mainly the tyrosine amino acids of the protein, although histidine can also be labelled (Fig. 2.1).

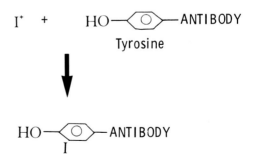

Fig. 2.1. Direct incorporation of radioiodine into antibody. Radioiodine as iodide is treated with an oxidising agent to give an intermediate I$^+$ which becomes covalently incorporated into amino acids in the protein structure, particularly into tyrosine.

Oxidizing agents used to promote the formation of cationic iodine can also have deleterious effects on the function of the monoclonal antibody being labelled by oxidizing various amino acid residues. Probably the extent of this will be a characteristic of the particular antibody being radiolabelled. There is no doubt that some antibodies are more robust than others. Although radiolabelling may be successful, the labelled preparation may have lost much of its immunological reactivity; hence with each antibody the chosen method of labelling must be shown not to compromise the reactivity of the antibody.

The radiolabelling of monoclonal antibodies for clinical use obviously requires the provision of the radioiodine from radiochemical manufacturers. Iodine-131 is widely available as a solution in sodium hydroxide at pH 7-11, free from reducing agent and specifically produced for protein iodination (for example, Amersham International supplies iodine-131 at up to 7.4 GBq/ml IBS30). Since iodination of monoclonal antibody is generally carried out on an individual patient basis, and activity in the range of 70-140 MBq of material is required, the volumes of the radioiodine solution used are very small (order of a few microlitres).

Iodine-123 is less readily available than iodine-131 and is not supplied in a radiochemical form specifically designed for protein iodination. This radionuclide has been little used in the USA for labelling monoclonal antibodies, mainly because of poor availability, although it is, of course, used for other radiopharmaceuticals such as MIBG. In Europe it is produced in the UK by the Atomic Energy Research Establishment, at Harwell in Switzerland by the Swiss Federal Institute for Reactor Research, and in Belgium by the National Institute for Radioelements, from whom it is available commercially from IRE-Med-

genix, Fleurus, Belgium. As will be discussed later, factors influencing the radioiodination of monoclonal antibodies include protein and radioiodine concentrations and reaction pH, and with iodine-123 preparations they may be of low concentration and/or require adjustment of pH.

Many different reagents and methods have been described for oxidative radioiodination of antibodies. Only those most frequently used for labelling antibodies for clinical administration will be described in detail here. Monoclonal antibody preparations for radiolabelling are usually produced at a concentration of several milligrams/ml. On a patient-by-patient basis it is usual to aim to produce between 70 and 140 MBq of labelled material containing 1–10 milligrams of antibody. Given that radioiodine is available at a high concentration, the iodination reaction volumes are usually small, often less than one millilitre. This has the advantages of maintaining high concentration of the monoclonal antibody (one factor influencing the efficiency of incorporation of radioiodine). The reaction vessel may be easily shielded and handled during the preparation and any subsequent purification steps.

The chloramine-T method. Chloramine-T is the sodium salt of N-chloro-p-toluene sulphonamide (Fig. 2.2). In aqueous solution it slowly produces hypochlorous acid and is therefore a mild oxidizing agent. For this method of labelling, antibody in solution buffered at pH 7 to 8 (the optimum for incorporation of iodine) is mixed with the radioiodine and an aqueous solution of freshly prepared chloramine-T added. This can be prepared at such concentration that only microlitre amounts need to be added to the reaction vessel, with minimal effects on the concentration of protein and radioiodine. Reaction times and conditions reported to have

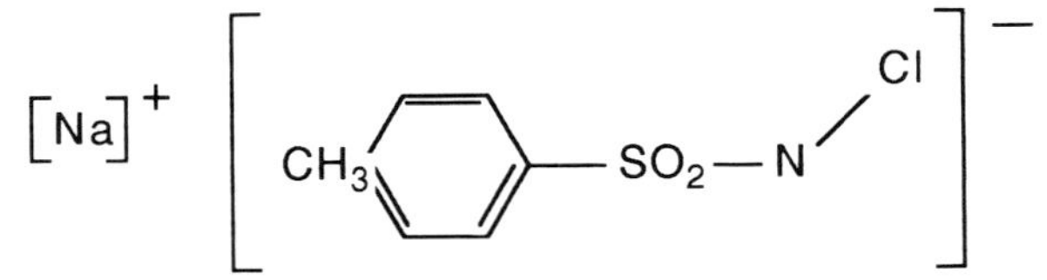

Fig. 2.2. Structure of chloramine-T, one of the most widely used oxidising agents used to catalyse incorporation of radioiodine into antibodies. The material is water soluble and is added to a solution of radioiodide and antibody. Its action has then to be stopped by the addition of a reducing agent.

been used for successful labelling of monoclonal antibodies for clinical use vary widely, but generally 10 to 20 μg of chloramine-T are used for each 37 MBq of radioiodine being used in the labelling of 0.5 to 1.0 mg of antibody. Reaction times also vary but are usually in the range of two to five minutes, usually at room temperature. The shorter the time, the less likely is oxidative damage to the antibody. The oxidative action of the chloramine-T is then usually stopped by the addition of an appropriate amount of a reducing agent. Sodium metabisulphite has often been used for this, although other reducing agents such as cysteine are also now being used. In some cases the reaction is stopped by the addition of excess tyrosine or tyramine, which will be iodinated at the expense of continuing iodination of the protein.

As an alternative to the use of chloramine-T as a solution, non-porous polystyrene beads coated with an immobilized form of the chemical are commercially available (IODO-BEADS™, Pierce Chemical Company). These beads are about ⅛th of an inch (3 mm) in diameter. Beads are added to the radioiodine solution about five minutes before the addition of antibody solution. The reaction can be stopped simply by removing the beads from the solution, and there is no need for the addition of reducing agent. Reaction conditions can be varied by the use of different numbers of beads, to achieve, for example, different specific activities, but

once standardized conditions have been set, the reaction is reported to be very reproducible. Although this method has been reported to have been used for radiolabelling monoclonal antibodies with iodine-125 for experimental use, it does not seem to have been widely used for clinical labelling with iodine-131 or iodine-123.

In some situations, particularly where small amounts of protein are being radiolabelled, it is usual to add carrier iodide and protein (e.g., 1% human serum albumin) to the reaction mixture to facilitate further purification of the labelled product. This is not generally regarded as necessary with the quantities of monoclonal antibody used for clinical studies, given the high radiolabelling efficiency usually achieved.

The iodogen method. Fraker and Speck (1978) introduced iodogen™ (Pierce Chemical Company) as an alternative to chloramine-T to minimize exposure of proteins to soluble oxidizing agents during radioiodination. Iodogen is probably now more widely used than chloramine-T. Chemically the material is 1,3,4,6,-tetrachloro-3α,6α-diphenylglycoluril (Fig. 2.3). It is virtually insoluble in water, and for protein iodination it is coated on the inner surface of the reaction vessel, by evaporation under a stream of nitrogen of a solution of the material in chloroform or methylene chloride. Small glass or solvent-resistant plastic (e.g., polypropylene) tubes capable of holding up to 1 or 2 ml of solution are ideal for this purpose. They can be prepared in large numbers and

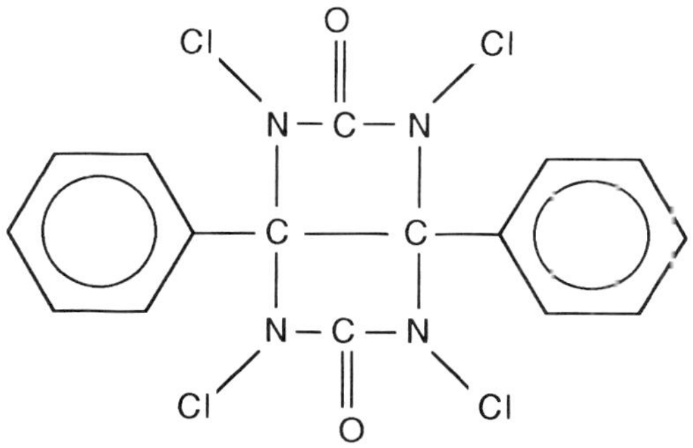

Fig. 2.3. Structure of Iodogen, now becoming more widely used than chloramine-T for oxidative incorporation of radioiodine into antibodies. This material is virtually insoluble in water and is usually coated onto the walls of reaction vessels for iodination. The reaction with radioiodide and antibody can be terminated simply by removing the solution from the vessel.

stored refrigerated for many months. Iodination reactions are then carried out by adding the appropriate volume of monoclonal antibody solution buffered to pH 7–8 and radioiodine to the coated tube, mixing, and leaving, usually at room temperature, for two to five minutes. The reaction is then stopped simply by removing the reaction solution from the tube. It is not usual to add carrier protein or iodide to the reaction mixture removed from the reaction tube. As with the iodogen method, some reactive species of iodide are thought to be still present in the solution even after removal from the reaction tube, and these could label carrier protein unless sufficient time (15 minutes) has elapsed for their chemical decay.

As with chloramine-T, the efficiency of labelling depends upon the pH of the reaction (being optimal in the range 7 to 8) and on the concentration of the antibody being labelled. Labelling efficiencies of generally greater than 60% and often 90% can be achieved. The amount of iodogen coated onto the surface of the reaction tube varies in published reports, but it is generally in the range 2 to 50 µg for clinical scale iodin-

ations. Smooth coating over the surface from evaporation of small (up to 1 ml) volumes of solution is difficult to achieve, and therefore not all of the iodogen may be available for reaction. This could be a limitation to achieving reproducibly high efficiency of radioiodine incorporation. To overcome this problem, an alternative method for the use of iodogen has been proposed (Richardson et al., 1986). This also seems particularly suitable for high efficiency radioiodination of lower concentrations of monoclonal antibodies and/or where radioiodine, such as iodine-123, may not be available at high concentration. In this technique a fine suspension of iodogen is produced by adding a small volume of a concentrated solution of the material in acetone to phosphate-buffered saline at pH 7 to 8. The iodogen comes out of solution to give a suspension of 3 µm diameter particles, an appropriate volume of which is then added to the mixture of monoclonal antibody and radioiodine. Over 90% efficiency of labelling antibody preparation by this technique have been reported. As with all of these iodination reactions involving oxidative incorporation into protein, the optimum pH range of the reaction was 7 to 8. The amount of iodogen added was 5 mol/mol antibody to give high (greater than 85%) incorporation of radioiodine. Presumably when monoclonal antibody preparations labelled in this way are for clinical use, the purification process to remove unreacted iodine will also remove the particulate iodogen from the preparation (see below).

The N-bromosuccinimide method. An alternative oxidizing agent recently proposed for use in the radioiodination of monoclonal antibodies is N-bromosuccinimide (Mather and Ward, 1987). This is water-soluble and is added in solution directly to the antibody/radioiodine mixture. Efficiencies of radioiodine incorporation, at least at high protein concentrations, are well over 90%, and the method has been introduced to achieve high specific labelling of antibody preparations for radioimmunotherapeutic rather than diagnostic use. With such high efficiency of incorporation, there may not be a need for a purification step to remove unreacted radioiodine, thus reducing radiation dose to the operator. This does mean that the N-bromosuccinimide present in the labelled preparation is ultimately administered to the patient, although the dose potentially given is insignificant as far as the known toxicity of the material is concerned. Simple purification steps used to remove unreacted radioiodine would also remove this material.

Other methods. A number of other techniques have been used for direct incorporation of radioiodine into proteins, including antibodies (Eckelman et al., 1980). Their use has rarely extended to clinical labelling of monoclonal antibodies, perhaps because of technical difficulties in the radiopharmacy setting, cost, or efficiency of incorporation of the radioiodine, although such methods are used in experimental situations and for radiolabelling antibodies for radioimmunoassays. For example, the enzyme lactoperoxidase, in the presence of hydrogen peroxide, catalyses the incorporation of radioiodine into tyrosine amino acids of proteins. This method of radiolabelling has been used to label monoclonal antibodies for biodistribution studies in experimental animals and would be suitable perhaps for labelling monoclonal antibodies difficult to radiolabel by any of the other methods, particularly where problems with immunological reactivity of the labelled preparations are encountered.

Indirect labelling. There are a number of techniques available, and others being developed, for the indirect labelling of monoclonal antibodies. There are a num-

ber of potential advantages in the use of these techniques. Firstly, the antibody is not exposed to the oxidizing conditions necessary for all of the direct iodination methods, nor to the reducing agents used in some techniques, such as the chloramine-T method. Some monoclonal antibodies are certainly damaged by these oxidation conditions, and indirect labelling may produce labelled antibody of higher immunoreactivity. Secondly, although as will be discussed later, the metabolism of monoclonal antibodies, particularly when they have reacted *in vivo* with target antigen, is as yet poorly understood, there is evidence that radioiodinated antibodies can undergo a process of de-iodination, usually referred to as dehalogenation. An obvious consequence of this is removal of the radioiodine from antibody which may have localised on, say, a tumour. Introduction of the radioiodine by a different chemical linkage, rather than incorporation into the tyrosine residues of the antibody, may give slower release of the label at *in vivo* sites, resulting in higher or more prolonged target to non-target ratios. Finally, some of these indirect techniques are being aimed at site-specific labelling of antibody molecules, particularly to label the Fc portion of the molecule. This positions the radioiodine atoms well away from the antigen-combining site of the molecule, potentially leaving the antibody in a highly immunoreactive form and possibly favourably altering the *in vivo* catabolism of the antibody. Although these techniques are only at the research stage and have not yet been introduced into clinical trials, it is expected that future developments in radioiodinated antibodies will take this form.

One of the earliest of these indirect labelling methods was that proposed by Bolton and Hunter (1973). Here 3-(4-hydroxyphenyl)propionic acid N-hydroxysuccinimide ester (now known as Bolton

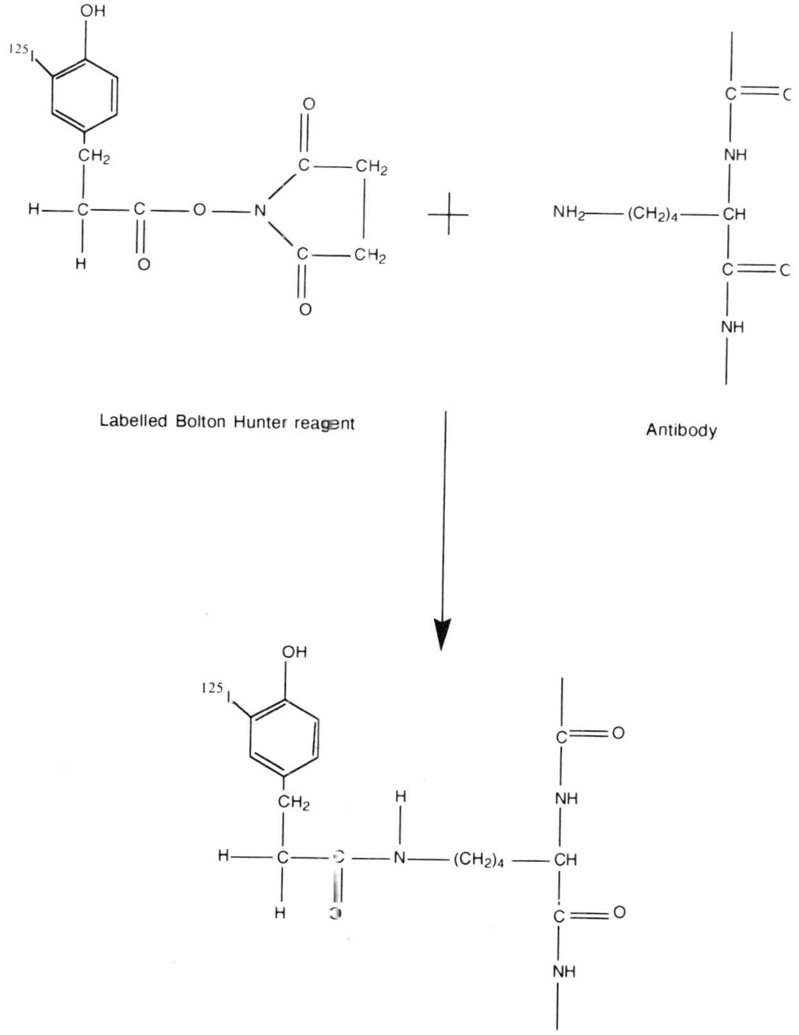

Labelled Antibody

Fig. 2.4. Indirect incorporation of radioiodine into antibody. Here 3-(4-hydroxyphenyl) propionic acid N-hydroxysuccinimide ester (known as Bolton and Hunter reagent) is first iodinated, using for example the chloramine-T or iodogen method, purified from the reactants, and then reacted with antibody. The reaction is the formation of an amide bond with the lysine groups of the antibody molecule. This method has been used most widely to label antibodies with iodine-125, and iodine-125 labelled Bolton and Hunter reagent is available for that purpose. The technique could also be adapted for iodine-131 labelling, although at present iodine-131-labelled reagent is not generally available commercially.

and Hunter reagent) is first iodinated, using, for example, the chloramine-T or iodogen method, purified from the reactants, and then reacted with antibody (Fig 2.4). During the reaction an amide bond is formed with the lysine groups of the antibody molecule. This method has been used most widely to label antibodies with iodine-125, and indeed iodine-125 labelled Bolton and Hunter reagent is available specifically for that purpose. The technique could also be adapted for iodine-131 labelling, although at present iodine-131-labelled reagent is not generally available commercially.

Another indirect labelling method currently being developed involves conjugating to the antibody cellobiose (a disaccharide of glucose) which has been conjugated to radioiodine labelled tyramine. Tyramine is the decarboxylated form of tyrosine and can be labelled with radioiodine by the chloramine-T or iodogen methods. Studies in experimental animals have shown higher and more prolonged retention of radioiodine in tumours using this labelling method compared with direct labelling with chloramine-T or lactoperoxidase.

Further refinements of indirect labelling are recently reported studies to introduce the radioiodine into the carbohydrate part of the antibody molecule. Carbohydrate is restricted to the Fc portion of the antibody molecule at a site distal to the antigen-combining site. One way to achieve labelling at the carbohydrate site is to oxidise the oligosaccharide to give free potentially reactive aldehyde groups, and to then conjugate to these a synthetic penta-peptide, glycyl-tyrosyl-glycyl-glycylarginine in which the tyrosyl group has been labelled with radioiodine. Studies in experimental animals with human tumour xenografts by Rodwell et al. (1986) using this method of labelling a monoclonal antibody showed

nearly twenty times as much radioiodine in tumour tissue compared with antibody labelled conventionally. Although most normal organs and the blood also showed higher levels of radioiodine, overall the discrimination between tumour and normal tissues was increased.

Purification of radiolabelled preparations. Some of the radioiodination methods described above can give nearly 100% incorporation of iodine into the monoclonal antibody. However, in practice it is usual to purify the preparation before final membrane filtration, dilution, and clinical administration. Radiopharmaceutical companies producing monoclonal antibodies labelled with I-131 will probably supply them already labelled and with free I-131 removed, and therefore suitable for patient administration. If antibodies have to be labelled in the radiopharmacy —and with I-123 this will usually be the case—it may be necessary to remove free radioiodine. The most widely used and simple technique here is gel filtration, and Sephadex® (Pharmacia) G25 or G50 is most commonly used. Because the volume from the labelling reaction is small (usually no more than 1 ml), only small columns of Sephadex are needed for efficient separation of protein from free radioiodide. Small pre-packed columns of Sephadex G25 are available and contain 0.05% Merthiolate®, which is a bactericide. The columns should be washed prior to use with sterile saline. Because of the small size of these columns and the fact that often milligram quantities of antibody are being labelled, there is rarely need to add carrier protein (e.g., human serum albumin) to prevent non-specific binding to the fabric of the column. The mixture from the labelling reaction is added to the top of the column and eluted from the column by addition of saline for injection to the column. The pre-packed columns have a surface tension net at the

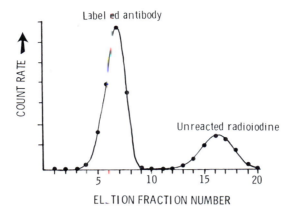

Fig. 2.5. Separation of unreacted radioiodine from labelled antibody. Here the reaction mixture of radioiodine and a monoclonal antibody which had been withdrawn from a reaction vessel coated with iodogen were passed through a small column of Sephadex G25 eluted in sterile saline. The labelled antibody flows straight through the column and appears in the first peak of eluted radioiodine. Unreacted radioiodine is retarded by the Sephadex and is eluted later.

top of the gel so that the liquid can only drop to the top of the gel bed (the column cannot run dry), and addition of, say, 0.5 ml of saline to the top is followed by simultaneous elution of the same volume from the bottom. Thus small fractions can easily be eluted from the column into a series of sterile containers and the amount of radioiodine assayed in a radionuclide calibrator. The labelled antibody elutes first from the column, and the free radioiodine comes off later (Fig. 2.5). Efficiencies of labelling may then be calculated from the input amount of radioiodine and that recovered in the labelled antibody fractions.

To examine labelled preparations for free radioiodine, either immediately after labelling, or after further purification, there are a number of simple techniques available. Most of these depend on the rapid denaturation and precipitation of proteins in highly acidic conditions. For this a trace of the labelled preparation can be diluted into a convenient volume, say 0.5 ml, containing approximately 10% human serum albumin, and a 20% solution of trichloracetic acid (TCA) in water added

to make the solution 10% with respect to TCA. The carrier albumin and the monoclonal antibody will be rapidly precipitated. Centrifugation can be used to separate the precipitate from supernatant, and radioiodine measured in the pelleted precipitate and in the supernatant. A more rapid refinement of this procedure, and one not requiring the addition of carrier protein, is to spot the labelled material near the bottom edge of a small strip (1 × 10 cm) of filter paper, and stand the paper with its bottom in a 10% solution of TCA to produce a simple ascending chromatogram. The paper strip can then be cut, and radioiodine remaining at the origin, due to acid precipitation of the protein-bound material, and that ascending with the solvent front (i.e., the free radioiodine), determined. A similar technique has been described using pre-prepared commercially available instant thin-layer chromatography strips and using 85% methanol to produce an ascending chromatogram.

Efficiencies of radioiodine incorporation can vary widely, depending on the labelling technique used and particularly on the protein concentration; the higher this is, the greater the efficiency usually achieved. Efficiencies approaching 100% are reported in some instances such as with the N-bromosuccinimide method described earlier, obviating the need for purification. Where purification methods are used to separate unreacted radioiodine, the proportion of antibody-bound iodine in the materials usually reported are in excess of 90%, and are usually in the range of 95–100%. The specific activities of radioiodine labelled antibodies used in clinical imaging studies is usually in the range of 37 to 370 MBq/mg of antibody protein. The dose of radioiodine used is usually 70–80 MBq for iodine-131, although with iodine-123 the dose may be higher, and up to 300 MBq have been used in some imaging studies.

Antibody Labelling
With Radioindium

Direct stable labelling of monoclonal antibodies with radiometals such as indium-111 is not possible without adversely effecting the immunological function of the antibody. Radiolabelling is generally achieved by pre-conjugation to the antibody of a chelating agent whose negatively charged carboxyl groups will subsequently bind by ionic interaction to the positively charged indium ions.

The first chelating agent introduced for this by Krejcarek and Tucker in 1977 was a mixed carboxycarbonic anhydride of diethyltriaminepentaacetic acid (DTPA). The anhydride interacts with amino groups of protein to form stable covalent amide bonds and can then be used to chelate indium ions. This procedure has been used in a number of clinical imaging trials, and was used in one of the first reports of imaging with indium-111 labelled antibody, using an anti-myosin antibody in experimental myocardial infarction in dogs (Khaw et al., 1980). However, the synthesis of the mixed anhydride is complex, it is unstable, and only low coupling efficiencies were achieved. Consequently Hnatowich et al. (1983a) introduced another anhydride of DTPA, a bicyclic anhydride (Fig. 2.6). This was more stable and soon became commercially available, and is now probably more widely used than the mixed anhydride. Hnatowich et al. (1983b) and also Richardson et al. (1987) have described conditions for optimization of DTPA anhydride (DTPAA) conjugation to antibodies and the preparation of DTPA-labelled antibody kits for routine use in indium-111 labelling for immunoscintigraphy. Other chelating agents are being developed for antibody labelling, particularly benzyl-EDTA and benzyl-TETA (Cole et al., 1987), but these have not yet reached a stage suitable for routine clinical use, and the bicyclic anhydride of DTPA is probably the most widely evaluated chelator at the present time.

To prevent hydrolysis of the DTPA anhydride, it has to be kept dry, and in the early work it was added to the antibody solution as a solid. However, because such small amounts of anhydride are needed to give the required molar ratio of anhydride to antibody, it would be impractical to weigh such a small amount, and often the anhydride was dried down into the reaction vessel from solution in anhydrous chloroform. However, because of the difficulty in achieving uniformly dried films of the material, the subsequent reaction with antibody was very variable. This could lead to variation in the ability of the DTPA-conjugated antibody to subsequently chelate indium. Consequently, a much simpler and reproducible way of reacting DTPAA with the antibody was developed. Here the DTPAA is dissolved in anhydrous dimethylsulphoxide, and the required volume

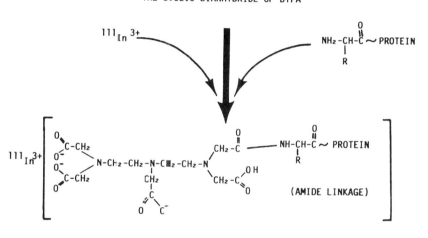

DTPA

THE CYCLIC DIANHYDRIDE OF DTPA

CHELATION OF ^{111}In

Fig. 2.6. Labelling of antibody with radioindium. DTPA is converted to its cyclic dianhydide (now commercially available), and this reacted with the antibody to give a stable antibody-DTPA conjugate which can subsequently chelate radioindium

added in a series of small aliquots to the antibody solution with continual stirring. Dimethylsulphoxide is miscible with aqueous solutions, and gives a much smoother and more reproducible reaction with the antibody before material which has not reacted with the antibody is hydrolysed to free DTPA.

Optimum pH conditions for the reaction of DTPAA with antibody are within the range of 7 to 9. Antibody available in routine phosphate-buffered saline at pH 7.2

can be used, but the reaction will be somewhat more efficient if the pH is increased to 8.0 by the addition of 0.5 M sodium bicarbonate. If antibody solution is available at a concentration of several milligrams/ml, conjugation efficiencies are high using the DMSO solution of DTPAA method. To achieve a 1:1 ratio of DTPA to antibody, probably the optimum for most indium-111 labelling requirements, an input ratio of 2 or 3:1 is used. Unreacted DTPA can then be removed from the reaction mixture either by gel filtration, using, for example, Sephadex G25, or dialysis, and the antibody-DTPA conjugate may be returned to phosphate-buffered saline. Antibody-DTPA preparations can be processed by centrifugation, filtration, sterility and pyrogen testing, etc. at this stage and dispensed into aliquots which may be stored suitable for individual patient studies (see Chapter 1, this volume). Storage conditions vary: certainly some antibody-DTPA conjugates can be stored refrigerated without loss of activity for many months, although some are stored frozen at $-20°C$ or $-80°C$.

Subsequent radiolabelling of antibody-DTPA conjugates is carried out by the addition of indium-111. This is usually available in radiopharmaceutical quality, as a solution of indium chloride, but this is not suitable for addition directly to the antibody-DTPA. Chelation of the radioindium takes place most efficiently at pHs below 5; however, to prevent the formation of colloidal forms of the indium it is necessary to add acetate or citrate to the reaction mixture. It is advisable to add an equal volume of 0.1 M sodium acetate, or citrate at pH 5, to the solution of indium chloride before its addition to the antibody. Alternatively, the antibody-DTPA conjugate can be prepared in 0.3 M citrate buffer at pH 6 during gel filtration or dialysis purification following reaction with the DTPA anhydride. Under these conditions, radio-indium can be directly added to the antibody-DTPA conjugate without any pretreatment, and this method is therefore technically the most simple. The reaction volumes during the labelling process need only be small, with the required amount of antibody-DTPA in probably less than 1 ml, and this allows the mixing of the indium and antibody-DTPA in the indium delivery vessel. Labelling efficiencies approaching 100% are often possible. For a 80 MBq patient dose of indium-111-labelled antibody, about 100 MBq per labelling procedure is usually sufficient to give the required dose after filtration and dilution, etc.

Purification of radioindium labelled preparations. Labelling of antibody-DTPA conjugates with indium-111 can be virtually 100% efficient, and obviously radiopharmaceutical companies producing kits for immunoscintigraphy will produce them in such a form that simple addition of In-111 as indium chloride is all that is necessary. In the developmental stages, though, with a new antibody or new DTPA conjugation procedure, it is advisable to remove any free indium. This can be carried out by small-scale gel filtration as outlined above for the purification of radioiodine labelled preparations. The amount of free indium-111 in preparations before or after purification is most easily measured by silica gel thin-layer chromatography. Here samples of the preparation are spotted onto the gel plate and eluted by ascending solvent consisting of one part 0.5 M citric acid:two parts 10% ammonium formate:two parts methanol. Antibody-bound indium remains at the origin, while unbound migrates with the solvent front. Assay of the activity of each portion will give the proportion of the total amount bound to antibody.

Determination of the molar ratio of DTPA:antibody in the conjugates is most conveniently carried out at the DTPA conjugation stage, before the unreacted DTPA has been removed from the reaction mixture. This relies on the distribution of indium between free and protein-bound DTPA. A small amount of radioindium is added to the antibody:DTPA anhydride mixture before removal of unreacted DTPA and the percentage of indium present as labelled protein determined. Because free and coupled DTPA compete equally for radioindium, the percentage of the added radioindium which is bound to the protein is equal to the coupling efficiency of the reaction of the DTPA anhydride with the antibody. The average number of DTPA groups attached per antibody molecule may be obtained from the coupling efficiency and the initial anhydride:protein molar ratio (Hnatowich et al., 1983b). Coupling efficiencies vary with antibody and DTPA anhydride concentrations. The higher the molar ratio of DTPA to antibody in the preparation, the more efficient will be subsequent chelation of the radioindium. However, as will be described later, the immunological reactivity of the antibody is often reduced by addition of more than two or three DTPA groups per molecule.

Antibody Labelling With Technetium-99m

As we have seen above, there are now relatively simple methods available for labelling of monoclonal antibodies with radioiodine and with radioindium. Radiolabelling with technetium to give products suitable for *in vivo* imaging is now also reaching this stage. Numerous methods of labelling proteins with technetium have been described. The main problem with some of these is that they rely on direct binding to the protein to stabilise the reduced technetium, thus preventing reoxidization to pertechnetate and the formation of colloidal technetium. Because of the wide use of technetium in nuclear med-

icine, there has been an enormous amount of commercial interest (and effort) to produce a reliable and simple method for radiolabelling antibody with this radionuclide. Some of the more effective methods for labelling monoclonal antibodies with technetium have been prepared in the form of kits available from commercial manufacturers. It is difficult to judge the relative merits of the different methods in terms of the quality of the product and the final images. This is mainly because there are little comparative data using the same antibody system radiolabelled with the different techniques. Methods reported in the literature are generally more complex than those with radioiodine or radioindium, and some procedures that have been described seem too complex for the average radiopharmacy to apply to monoclonal antibodies in their native form.

The methods described for technetium labelling of antibodies fall into two broad groups. Firstly, there are those requiring initial attachment to the antibody of a chelator which will subsequently bind the technetium. Secondly, there are those which require modification of the antibody protein itself to allow subsequent binding of the technetium. Most, but not all, require the reduction of pertechnetate (TcO_4^-), produced from technetium generators, to a cationic form of technetium (Tc^{4+}). The favourable patient dosimetry of technetium-99m means that higher doses of this radionuclide than radioiodine or radioindium can be used, often up to 1000 MBq. If the amount of antibody protein to be administered is not to be increased beyond one or two milligrams used for radioiodine or radioindium labelled preparations, this means that the specific activity of technetium-99m labelled preparations will be much higher than that of the other preparations.

Bifunction chelating methods. Based on the successful use of DTPA for labelling monoclonal antibodies with radioindium, Childs and Hnatowich (1985) investigated this method for labelling with technetium. DTPA was conjugated to the antibody by reaction with its anhydride. Stannous chloride was used to reduce the pertechnetate by first adding the tin salt to the antibody. Stannous ions themselves are chelated by the DTPA on the antibody, and when pertechnetate was subsequently added, all three reactants (i.e., the stannous ion, the pertechnetate, and the DTPA) were in close proximity during the reduction process in the hope of favouring labelling of DTPA rather than non-specific sites on the protein. Although this method does produce labelled antibody with immunological reactivity and *in vivo* stability better than that of antibody labelled only by non-specific binding to the protein, it has not been possible to reduce to negligible levels the degree of non-specific binding. Although monoclonal antibodies labelled in this way have been used in some experimental systems—for example, in tumour localization and imaging—the method does not seem to have been used in many clinical studies.

An alternative chelating agent has more recently been described by Arano et al. (1986). This uses a new bifunctional chelating agent containing a di(N-methylthiosemicarbazone) as the technetium coordinating site and an aralkyl carboxylate site for protein conjugation. So far this method has not been reported to have been used to label monoclonal antibodies, but in model studies with human serum albumin, a product with high *in vivo* stability was obtained.

Another method of chelating technetium to antibodies, which has been examined by Brown et al. (1988), is to first attach the antibody, using a bifunctional cross-linking agent, the small-molecular-weight metal binding protein metallo-

thionein. Following purification the metallothionein-antibody conjugate can be labelled with reduced technetium. Although used in experimental studies, the method has not yet been used clinically, although labelling of anti-tumour monoclonal antibodies was successful with this method.

Direct labelling methods. It is now known that exposure of antibodies to reduction with, for example, stannous ions reduces some of the disulphide bonds in the protein structure, producing free thiol groups, and that these can react with reduced technetium (Rhodes et al., 1986). This requires careful control of the reduction conditions, as the labelling involves the interposition of the technetium atoms between the heavy chains of the antibody molecule, and if not carried out carefully, the antibody may be fragmented. This approach has been developed for the production of kits for labelling monoclonal antibodies with technetium-99m (Schwarz and Steinstrasser, 1987). Here the antibody is reduced using a thiol such as 2-mercaptoethanol or 2-aminoethanethiol and is then freeze dried. For labelling, the antibody is reconstituted and reacted with pertechnetate reduced with stannous salt. This method of labelling has been used in a number of centres for clinical imaging and has been adopted for the preparation of imaging kits now becoming commercially available. Mather et al. (1990) have investigated the use of this technique and found it suitable for a number of different antibodies. The procedure involved first concentrating the antibody to approximately 10 mg per ml. The material is then reduced for 30 minutes at room temperature with 2-mercaptoethanol at a molar ratio of 1000 to 1 and purified by Sephadex G50 gel filtration. The antibody fractions can then be aliquoted and stored at $-20°C$ prior to radiolabelling. The radiolabelling is carried

out by adding 0.2 ml of a methylene diphos-
phonate bone scanning kit reconstituted
with 5 ml normal saline, followed by up to
1200 MBq (30 mCi) Tc-99m. The product
may then be purified by passing through a
Sephadex G50 column using 1% HSA/PBS
solution.

An alternative method of directly labelling antibody with technetium-99m has
been recently described, although the exact mechanism of the labelling chemistry
has not yet been clarified. Here pertechnetate is treated with dimethylformamide
and hydrochloric acid at high temperature
(140°C) for 4 hours. The reaction product
is dissolved in chloroform and appropriate
amounts dried down by evaporation before
antibody solution is added. It is thought
that the reaction which then takes place
between the technetium-labelled intermediate and the protein involves coupling at
the amino groups of the protein. Experimentally the technique has been used to
label anti-fibrin and anti-renal cell carcinoma antibodies (Dijk et al., 1988).

A further method which has been reported is the use of a diamide dimercap-
tide (N$_2$S$_2$) ligand. This forms highly stable
complexes with technetium. This can either be conjugated to the antibody and
then labelled with the radiolabel, or pre-
formed complexes can be conjugated to
the antibody (Frer et al., 1988; Serafini et
al., 1988). Clinically there are reports of
the use of this labelling method in imaging
lung carcinoma and melanoma.

Radiolabelling With Other Radionuclides

Gallium-67 has not been widely used for
labelling monoclonal antibodies for clinical imaging. In experimental studies it has
been used to label antibodies for imaging
tumours, and here the antibody was conjugated to DTPA, as for indium-111 labelling

and gallium-67 attached by chelation from
a solution of gallium citrate (Haisma et al.,
1984). An alternative method described by
Koizumi et al. (1987) involves conjugation
first to the antibody of deferoxamine,
which subsequently chelates gallium.

The choice of other radionuclides with
suitable half-lives, energies of gamma
emission, and patient dosimetry for use in
immunoscintigraphy is limited. The only
other radionuclide reported to be under
investigation is lead-203 with a half-life of
52 hours and gamma emission at 279 keV
(Srivastava et al., 1988).

PRODUCT HOMOGENEITY AND IMMUNOLOGICAL REACTIVITY

In many ways immunoradiopharmaceuticals are easier to characterise than standard radiopharmaceuticals. This is mainly
because the functional capability of the radiolabelled product may be measured by
reaction with the target antigen.

When monoclonal antibodies have been
radiolabelled, it is relatively easy to determine the amount of radionuclide in the
preparation which is attached to the antibody protein. As outlined above, this can
be done by simple precipitation tests or
small scale chromatographic techniques.
These tests will not, however, give information about the homogeneity of the labelled preparation nor about the immunological reactivity of the labelled antibody
molecules. It is crucial to assess the characteristics of the radiolabelled preparations, because the labelling process itself
may cause aggregation of the antibody molecules, which will alter the *in vivo* biodistribution pattern and prevent effective localization on the target antigen, or it may
damage the antigen binding site of the antibody which will limit reaction with the
target antigen. Although it is probably not
necessary to carry out tests to determine

the homogeneity and immunological reactivity of each individual antibody dose, these tests should be done as routine quality control on samples from each batch of antibody before it is regarded as suitable for release for experimental or clinical use.

These quality control measures should be regarded as standard techniques used in conjunction with the other standard QC procedures associated with good radiopharmacy practice. Although these procedures are relatively new in the context of the radiopharmacy, the techniques which have been most widely used to examine the homogeneity of labelled preparations include standard biochemical/immunological methods.

Homogeneity of Preparations

SDS-polyacrylamide gel electrophoresis is well established for determining molecular weights of proteins, including antibodies and their fragments. High-performance liquid chromatography, with appropriate columns, is also widely used for protein size analysis. This has the advantage over SDS-PAGE in that it will also detect free, non-protein-bound radiolabel—for example, In-111 complexed to free DTPA. In the absence of these techniques, gel filtration chromatography on media such as Sephadex® G-200 or Sephacryl® S-300 (Pharmacia) can be employed. These columns can be calibrated with molecular weight markers, including IgG and antibody fragments, and any deviation from the expected molecular size of the labelled antibody or fragment will be seen. With this method it is often appropriate to add a sample of the labelled antibody to serum before the gel filtration run. This will itself give a calibration of the elution characteristics of the column, since the serum proteins will be fractionated into three regions, and with indium-111 as the radio-

label, any free indium will be taken up by the transferrin in the serum and run on the chromatographic separation quite distinctly from the labelled antibody (Fig. 2.7). In preparations used for clinical imaging it is usually reported that the majority (at least 90%) of the radiolabelled antibody or fragment is in its original monomeric form.

Immunological Reactivity

Indirect method. Assessment of the immunological reactivity of radiolabelled monoclonal antibody or fragment preparations is only possible if a convenient source of the target antigen is available. In some of these tests the immunological reactivity is assessed in an indirect method, similar to those used to test the target specificity of the monoclonal antibodies during their initial development. Here radiolabelled and parent unlabelled antibodies are reacted separately with target antigen, usually in a series of dilutions, and their binding then detected with an appropriately radio- or enzyme-labelled antibody against the mouse or human immunoglobulin of the monoclonal antibody under test. In this way the titre of labelled monoclonal antibody can be compared with that of the parent preparation. Unfortunately, the problem with this method is that it detects reactivity of all monoclonal antibody molecules in the preparation regardless of whether they are radiolabelled or not. With specific activities often used in clinical immunoscintigraphy (typical levels with radioiodines and radioindium are 80 MBq/mg), the majority of antibody molecules in the preparation may not actually be labelled, and it is possible to envisage a situation in which the radiolabelled molecules have lost most of their antigen binding capacity, but the presence of a larger amount of unlabelled and undamaged antibody molecules gives the impression that

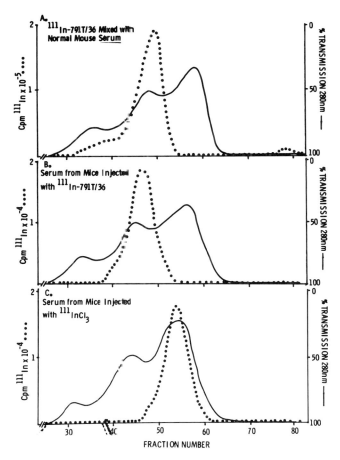

Fig. 2.7. Checking the homogeneity of labelled antibody by gel filtration chromatography. Here is an experimental study by the authors, In-111-labelled monoclonal antibody was added to mouse serum and chromatographed on Sephacryl S-300 (Panel A). Most of the radiolabeled eluted from the column as a discrete peak around fraction 48, co-incident with the second peak of protein resulting from the fractionation of the serum. Note however the shoulder on the ascending side of the peak indicative of some aggregated antibody, and the small peak of radioindium at fraction 80, indicative of a small amount of free radioindium or In-111-DTPA. The preparation was injected into mice and serum taken from them 48 hours later. The serum-borne radiolabel was now exclusively around fraction 48 indicating good survival of labelled antibody (Panel B) but clearance of aggregates and free radioindium. Contrast these with serum taken from mice after the injection simply of radioindium (as indium chloride) (Panel C). The serum-borne radioindium is now eluted around fraction 55, i.e., at a lower molecular weight, due to association of the radioindium with serum transferrin. (Reproduced from Perkins et al., Eur. J. Nucl. Med. 10:296–301, 1985, with permission of the publisher.)

the preparation as a whole has retained virtually full immunological reactivity. Obviously it is only the radiolabelled molecules which are detected during imaging, and really it is the immunological reactivity of these labelled molecules which needs to be assessed as part of the quality control of antibody preparations for immunoscintigraphy. Radiolabelled molecules which have lost their ability to react with target antigen will obscure imaging of those which have reacted with target antigen and will therefore lead to a reduction in target:non-target ratios.

Immunoreactive fraction. The immunological reactivity of the radiolabelled antibody or fragment molecules in a preparation can usually easily be determined by measuring the proportion of radiolabel in the preparation which can bind to target antigen. This proportion is usually referred to as the immunoreactive fraction of the labelled antibody preparation.

The conventional way to determine the immunoreactive fraction of a radiolabelled antibody preparation is to measure the highest fraction of the radiolabel count which can bind to target antigen in an assay set up where antigen is in excess over antibody so that there is antigen available for all of the immunoreactive antibody to bind to. This usually requires a titration with either a fixed amount of antigen and a series of dilutions of the antibody or a fixed amount of antibody with increasing amounts of antigen. The source and manner of presentation of the antigen will obviously depend on the nature of the antigen. For example, with antibodies against tumour-associated antigens, tumour cells grown in tissue culture and used as a freshly prepared viable cell suspension are frequently used. In some cases cells can be fixed with preservatives such as paraformaldehyde and stored awaiting assays. Cell membrane preparations can also be used. In the case of antibodies against some tumour associated antigens which are available in pure form, such as CEA, immunoabsorbants with the antigen attached to inert carriers such as Sepharose can be used. This latter method has also been used for monoclonal antibodies against fibrin where the fibrin was attached to Sepharose® (Pharmacia) (Rosebrough et al., 1988). It has also been suggested that anti-idiotypic antibody produced as a result of the immune response of subjects injected with the antibody may be used to measure immunoreactivity. The anti-idiotype essentially binds with the antibody in the same way as antigen.

These assays of immunological reactivity each need some negative controls, such as tumour target cell or antigen known not to react with the antibody under test. Inert carriers lacking antigen may also be used. Only in this way can it be shown that the binding of the radiolabelled material is actually an immunological process and is not due to non-specific "stickiness" of the labelled preparation. This phenomenon is always present to some extent with all antibody preparations and is likely to be increased with preparations damaged or aggregated during manipulations such as radiolabelling. Because radiolabelled preparations are normally tested at only low concentrations (often only ten's of nanograms/ml in order to ensure conditions of antigen excess), dilutions of antibodies should contain some added protein to prevent non-specific binding of the radiolabelled monoclonal antibody. Bovine serum albumin (BSA) at 1% in an appropriate buffer such as phosphate buffered saline at pH 7 is frequently used for this. The tests would usually consist of a series of replicates (two or three) of each dilution of the antibody/antigen mixture incubated for several hours with constant agitation. This incubation is often carried out at 4°C or at room temperature, but to stimulate *in vivo* conditions, may be carried out at 37°C. Tests with viable cell suspensions should best be carried out in the cold to prevent actual intracellular uptake of radiolabelled material by the cells in addition to the binding of cell surface antigens. Subsequently the antigen preparation is removed from the reaction, usually by centrifugation, and the proportion of the radiolabel bound determined by assay of the two components of the reaction, i.e., the antigen and the supernatant. Fig 2.8A shows an example of the binding of indium-111 labelled

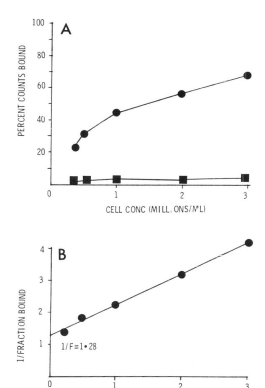

Fig. 2.8. Determining the immunoreactivity of radio-labelled antibody. Here in a study by the Authors an In-111 labelled anti-tumour antibody was tested for immunoreactivity by measuring the proportion of radiolabel which bound to tumour cells when increasing numbers of antigen positive (●) cells were incubated with a constant amount of antibody. The antibody did not bind to antigen negative cells (■) but showed increasing binding to increasing numbers of antigen positive cells. Although this was approaching 70% binding of the input counts a precise value cannot be determined (panel A). However when the same data is plotted as a double inverse plot (panel B) the points fall on a straight line. Extrapolation to the ordinate where 1/cell concentration = 0, i.e., a theoretical infinite number of cells, gives the 1/the fraction bound as 1.28, that is an immunoreactive fraction of 0.78, or 78%.

monoclonal antibody against tumour target cells. As the cell concentration increases, the proportion of radioindium binding to the cells increases, i.e., the reaction is tending to antigen excess so that all of the immunologically reactive antibody molecules have antigen available for binding. This example shows a highly immunologically reactive preparation, since the titration curve is reaching a plateau at about 80% of the input activity bound to the antigen-positive target cells and less than 5% to antigen-negative control cells. However, the exact plateau is difficult to determine from the plot as shown. A simple mathematical method of manipulating this sort of data has been described by Lindmo et al. (1984). This involves a double inverse plot of the total radioactivity applied over the amount of radioactivity bound as a function of the inverse cell concentration (Fig. 2.8B). By means of linear extrapolation to the ordinate, i.e., to where the inverse of the cell concentration is zero and to where the cell concentration is theoretically infinite, the immunoreactive fraction of the monoclonal antibody can be more accurately determined. This type of analysis has the advantage that it is quite insensitive to variations such as the actual concentration of cells (providing that the serial dilutions from the original are accurately made), the incubation time, the concentration of antibody, and the ratio of antigen to antibody used in the reaction. This technique was originally described using an anti-tumour monoclonal antibody with tumour cells as the target antigen, but can obviously be used with other forms of antigen; for example, increasing amounts of antigen-coated Sepharose could be used.

The immunoreactive fractions of radiolabelled monoclonal antibody or fragment preparations reported to have been used in clinical imaging vary widely, from as little as 10% to virtually 100%. It can be expected that the higher the immunoreactive fraction, the more efficient the imaging of target antigen. Clearly the highest possible immunoreactivity should be aimed for in any radiolabelled antibody preparation.

There is no doubt that antibody can lose its immune function if damaged during purification, fragmentation, or labelling. In the last of these contexts, some antibodies will be damaged by exposure to the oxidizing agents used in some radio-iodination procedures, and some may be damaged by attachment of too many chelating group used for subsequent chelation of radiometals.

It is possible to determine whether the immunoreactive fraction of a labelled preparation is a reflection of the intrinsic reactivity of the antibody preparation itself or whether it has been altered by the labelling procedure. For this purpose, binding assays against target antigen are set up under conditions where the antibody is clearly in excess over antigen. The proportion of radiolabel binding will be low, but if unlabelled native antibody is added to the reaction mixtures, it should quantitatively compete with the radiolabelled molecules for antigen sites. If an equal amount of labelled and unlabelled preparation are incubated with antigen, the proportion of the radiolabel which binds should be reduced by 50%.

Determination of the immunoreactive fraction of labelled preparations is essential before their clinical use to ensure that the particular antibody is being used in its optimum condition. Now that a wider range of monoclonal antibodies are becoming available, comparative imaging studies are clearly desirable to determine the relative diagnostic merits of these preparations. This can only be valid if all of the preparations are actually of more or less equal immunoreactivity. Commercially available radiolabelled monoclonal antibodies, and kits supplied ready for radiolabelling, should generally be of high immunoreactivity, with 80–90% of radiolabel binding to appropriate target antigen. Although not necessary on a routine basis, it would be desirable for manufacturers to supply appropriate antigen material to facilitate the measurement of immunoreactivity in the radiopharmacy should the need arise.

In addition to damage to monoclonal antibodies during purification or labelling, it is possible that some antibodies are intrinsically of low immunological reactivity, due to some defect in the parent hybridoma. If the hybridoma is grown ascitically in animals rather than in vitro culture, it may be damaged during prolonged in vivo exposure or become contaminated with the animal's normal immunoglobulin, both of which will affect the final immunoreactivity following purification. In these situations where antibody is of low immunoreactivity, it may be feasible to isolate the immunoreactive material by the use of specific immunoabsorbants, either before or after radiolabelling. Unfortunately, this adds to the complexity of the overall production techniques.

Antibody Affinity

Further analysis of data obtained during the determination of the immunoreactive fraction of the antibody or antibody fragment preparations can give a measure of the affinity of the binding to target antigen. In this case, the ratio of bound to free radiolabel is expressed as a function of the bound over a range of antigen-antibody incubation conditions. The amount of free, unbound, antibody is corrected for the immunoreactive fraction of the preparation so that only immunologically reactive material is considered in the calculation. The slope of a plot expressed in this way (the classical Scatchard plot) is a measure of the equilibrium constant (Ke) of the reaction of the antibody with target antigen

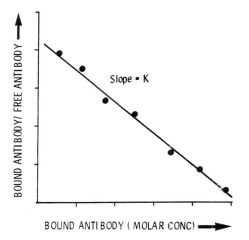

Fig. 2.9. Determining the affinity of radiolabelled antibody. The proportion of antibody specifically bound to target antigen is plotted against the molar concentration of bound antigen in a Scatchard plot. From consideration of the Law of Mass Action it can be shown that the slope of such a plot = Ke. Precisely measured concentrations of antibody are needed for this analysis and the concentration has to be expressed in terms of molarity. Furthermore the immunoreactive fraction of the antibody should also be determined because compensation has to be made for this in determining the amount of potentially reactive antibody still free.

(Fig. 2.9). This value is derived from the Law of Mass Action, which can be used to describe the equilibrium of the reaction of antigen with antibody

$$\text{Antibody} + \text{Antibody} \underset{\text{Kd}}{\overset{\text{Ka}}{\rightleftharpoons}}$$

$$\text{Antibody-Antigen}$$

by the equation

$$\text{Ke} = \text{Ka/Kd} = \frac{[\text{Antibody} - \text{Antigen}]}{[\text{Antigen}][\text{Antibody}]}$$

where Ke = equilibrium constant
Ka = the association constant
Kd = the dissociation constant

In this equation the concentration of the antigen and antibody is expressed in molar

concentrations, and the unit of the association constant is litres/mole. Typical Ke values for antibodies are in the range of 10^8–10^{11}. The higher the value, the higher the affinity of reaction of the antibody with antigen and therefore the better its potential interaction with target antigen *in vivo*. Clearly there is a desire for antibodies with affinities of 10^{11} or greater for efficient imaging.

Determination of the association constant of a monoclonal antibody radiolabelled in different ways, for example, by increasing the number of chelating groups per molecule or to higher specific activities, may reveal changes in the affinity of the radiolabelled molecules. In addition, changes in the immunoreactive fraction may be brought about by total destruction of antigen-binding capacity of some of the labelled molecules (Matzku et al., 1985).

Monoclonal antibodies selected for immunoscintigraphy should be of high intrinsic affinity and immunoreactivity, and these properties should be reduced as little as is practically possible following radiolabelling if their full potential is to be achieved.

REFERENCES AND FURTHER READING

Arano, Y., Yokoyama, A., Magata, Y., Saji, H., Horiuchi, K., Torizuka, K. (1986): Synthesis and evaluation of a new bifunctional chelating agent for 99m-Tc labelling proteins: p-carboxyethylphenylglyoxal-di(N-methylthiosemicarbazone). Int. J. Nucl. Med. Biol. 12:425–430.

Baum, R.P., Hertel, A., Lorenz, M., Schwarz, A., Encke, A., Hor, G. (1989): Immunoscintigraphy of known and occult metastatic colorectal carcinoma with Tc-99m-labelled anti-CEA monoclonal antibody for tumour immunoscintigraphy: First clinical results. Nucl. Med. Commun. 10:345–352.

Bolton A.E., Hunter, W.M. (1973): The labelling of proteins to high specific activity radioactivities by conjugation to a I-125 containing acylating agent. Biochem. Journal 133:529–538.

Brown, B.A., Drozynski, C.A., Deraborn, C.B., Hadjin, R.A., Liberatore, F.A., Tulip, T.A., Tolman, G.L.,

Haber, S.B. (1988): Conjugation of metallothionein to a monoclonal antibody. Anal. Biochem. 172:22–28.

Childs, R.L., Hnatowich, D.J. (1985): Optimum conditions for labelling of DTPA-coupled antibodies with technetium-99m. J. Nucl. Med. 26:293–299.

Cole, W.C., DeNardo, S.J., Meares, C.F., McCall, M.J., Denardo, G.L., Epstein, A.L., O'Brian, H.A., Moi, M.K. (1987): Comparative serum stability of radiochelates for antibody radiopharmaceuticals. J. Nucl. Med. 28:83–90.

Dijk, J.V., Oosterwijk, E., Kroonenburgh, M.J.P.G., Jonas, U., Fleuran, G.J., Pauwels, E.K.J., Warnaar, S.O. (1988): Perfusion of tumor bearing kidneys as a model for scintigraphic screening of monoclonal antibodies. J. Nucl. Med. 29:1078–1082.

Eckelman, W.C., Paik, C.H., Reba, R.C. (1980): Radiolabeling of antibodies. Cancer Res. 40: 3036–3042.

Fraker, P.J., Speck, J.C. (1978): Protein and cell membrane iodination with a sparingly soluble chloramide, 1,3,4,6-tetrachloro-3α,6α-diphenylglycoluril. Biochem. Biophys. Res. Commun. 80: 849–857.

Frer, M.F., Schroff, R.W., Abrams, P.G., Collins, C., Eary, J.F., Johnson, F., Lesley, T.M., Fritzberg, A.R., Nelp, W.C. (1988): Successful imaging of lung and colon carcinoma by a technetium-99m labeled monoclonal antibody. J. Nucl. Med. 29:834.

Haisma, H., Goedemans, W., Jong, M., Hilkens, J., Hilgers, J., Dullens, H., Den Otter, W. (1984): Specific localisation of indium-111 labeled monoclonal antibody versus Ga-67 labeled immunoglobulin in mice bearing human breast carcinoma xenografts. Cancer Immunol. Immunother. 17:62–65.

Hnatowich, D.J., Layne, W.W., Childs, R.L., Lanteigne, D., Davis, M.A., Griffen, T.W., Doherty, P.W. (1983a): Radioactive labelling of antibody: A simple and efficient method. Science 220: 613–615.

Hnatowich, D.J., Childs, R.L., Lantaigne, D., Najafi, A. (1983b): The preparation of DTPA-coupled antibodies radiolabeled with metallic radionuclides: An improved method. J. Immunol. Methods 65:147–157.

Hughes, W.L. (1957): The chemistry of iodination. Ann. N.Y. Acad. Sci. 70:3–17.

Khaw, B.A., Fallon, J.T., Strauss, H.W., Haber, E. (1980): Myocardial infarct imaging of antibodies to canine cardiac myosin with indium-111-diethylenetriamine pentaacetic acid. Science 209: 295–297.

Koizumi, M., Endo, K., Kunimatsu, M., Sakahara, H., Nakashima, T., Kawamura, Y., Watanabe, Y., Ohmomo, Y., Arano, Y., Yokoyama, A., Torizuka, K. (1987): Preparation of 67-Ga-labeled antibodies using deferoxamine as a bifunctional chelate. J. Immunol. Methods 104:93–102.

Krejcarek, G.E., Tucker, K.L. (1977): Covalent attachment of chelating groups to macromolecules.

Biochem. Biophys. Res. Commun. 77:581–585.

Lindmo, T., Boven, E., Cuttitta, F., Fedorko, J., Bunn, P.A. (1984): Determination of the immunoreactive fraction of radiolabelled monoclonal antibodies by linear extrapolation to binding at infinite antigen excess. J. Immunol. Methods 72:77–89.

Mather, S.J., Ward, B.C. (1987): High efficiency iodination of monoclonal antibodies for radiotherapy. J. Nucl. Med. 28:1034–1036.

Mather, S.J., Ellison, D. (1990): Reduction-mediated Technetium-99m labelling of monoclonal antibodies J. Nucl. Med. 31:692–697.

Matzku S., Kirchgessner H., Dippold, W.G., Bruggen, J. (1985): Immunoreactivity of monoclonal antimelanoma antibodies in relation to the amount of radioactive iodine substituted to the antibody molecule. Eur. J. Nucl. Med. 11:260–264.

Pimm, M.V., Baldwin, R.W. (1987): Comparative tumour localization properties of radiolabelled monoclonal antibody preparations of defined immunoreactivities. Eur. J. Nucl. Med. 13:348–352.

Rhodes, B.A., Zamora, P.O., Newall, K.D., Valdez, E.F. (1986): Technetium-99m labeling of murine monoclonal antibody fragments. J. Nucl. Med. 27:685–693.

Richardson, A.P., Mountford, P.J., Baird, A.C., Heyderman, E., Richardson, T.C., Coakley, A.J. (1986): An improved iodogen method of labelling antibodies with 123-I. Nucl. Med. Commun. 7:355–362.

Richardson, A.P., Mountford, P.J., Heyderman, E., Coakley, A.J. (1987): Optimization and batch production of DTPA-labelled antibody kits for routine use in indium-111 immunoscintigraphy. Nucl. Med. Commun. 8:347–365.

Rodwell, J.D., Alvarez, V.L., Lee, C., Lopes, A.D., Goers, J.W.F., King, H.D., Powsner, H.J., McKearn, T.J. (1986): Site-specific site covalent modification of monoclonal antibodies: In vitro and in vivo evaluations. Proc. Natl. Acad. Sci. (USA) 83:2632–2636.

Rosebrough, S.F., Grossman, Z.D., McAfee, J.G., Kudryk, B.J., Subramanian, G., Ritter-Hrncirik, C.A., Witanowski, L.S., Tillapaugh-Fay, G., Urrutia, E., Zapf-Longo, C. (1988): Thrombus imaging with indium-111 and iodine-131 labeled fibrin specific monoclonal antibody and its F(ab')2 and Fab fragment. J. Nucl. Med. 29:1212–1222.

Schwarz, A., Steinstrasser, A. (1987): A novel approach to Tc-99m-labeled monoclonal antibodies. J. Nucl. Med. 28:721.

Serafini, A.N., Kotler, J., Feun, L., Heal, A., Dewanjee, M., Friden, A., Abrams, P. (1988): Tc-99m labeled monoclonal antibodies in the detection of metastatic melanoma. Clinical experience in a phase III study. J. Nucl. Med. 29:897.

Srivastava, S.C., Meinken, G.E., Mease, R.C., Mausner, L.F., Steplewski, Z. (1988): Lead-203 as a new antibody label for radioimmunoimaging. J. Nucl. Med. 29:924.

3 Role of Animal Models for the Pre-Clinical Evaluation of Antibody Preparations

INTRODUCTION

In vitro hybridoma technology has produced a range of monoclonal antibodies against a number of antigens associated with human pathological lesions and which have, therefore, potential for *in vivo* localization and consequently could be exploited for diagnosis by immunoscintigraphy. Given that these monoclonal antibodies can be purified, can pass whatever toxicological testing the prevailing legislation requires, and can be satisfactorily labelled with appropriate radionuclides for clinical imaging, how can they be evaluated pre-clinically for imaging efficacy as part of the justification for clinical trials?

Obviously no animal model is ideal for human disease nor for understanding the biodistribution, catabolism, etc., of pharmaceutical agents. This is probably particularly so with antibodies. Most monoclonal antibodies currently available are of murine origin. Even before the advent of monoclonal antibodies, there was a large body of information about the biodistribution and catabolism of mouse, human, and other immunoglobulins of different classes and isotypes in their respective species of origin (Waldman and Strober, 1969; Covell et al., 1986). Although some mouse monoclonal antibodies have been evaluated in other species, including guinea pigs, dogs, and monkeys, the majority of animal biodistribution studies with these antibodies, as models for their clinical use, have been in mice with artificially induced target lesions. Clearly it is the pharmacokinetics of the antibodies that influence their ability to localize in the target lesion and to discriminate between it and normal tissue. But we cannot expect these mouse immunoglobulins, such as monoclonal antibodies, to behave pharmacokinetically when injected into man in quite the same as they do in mice, or even as they do in other species. The mouse antibody is a foreign protein in man, and although of very similar basic structure to human antibodies, it will not behave like human immunoglobulin when administered to patients. The two great differences between human and mouse antibodies when injected into patients are the much shorter plasma half-time of mouse IgG (usually of the order of one or two days compared with about twenty days for human IgG) and the ability of mouse antibodies as foreign proteins to evoke the production of immune responses, particularly antibodies, by the patients.

A further problem with animal models for immunoscintigraphy is that the target lesions may not be truly representative of the clinical situation because this model lesion will almost always have been artificially induced. This is particularly true with imaging of experimental tumours.

In spite of the limitations of experimental models, it has been the positive results from animal studies that have encouraged clinical evaluation and led to the present state of the art. Antibodies, particularly monoclonal antibodies, have been produced against antigens associated with a range of pathological conditions. Animal models have been developed for most of these conditions for the pre-clinical evaluation of these antibodies, most particularly to determine the imaging capability of the antibodies labelled with appropriate radionuclides. In addition, these model systems have been valuable in understanding some of the seemingly anomalous findings from clinical immunoscintigraphy.

TUMOUR LOCALISATION

Much of the early work on tumour localization of radiolabelled antibodies was carried out with antibodies against rodent tumours. Indeed these systems were the first to be used by Pressman and his colleagues in the 1950s in the original demonstration of the feasibility of localizing antibodies in tumours (Pressman and Korngold, 1953). These animals have the limitation, however, that their tumours are not suitable models for the corresponding human malignancies since antibodies raised against, for example, human colorectal carcinoma do not react with animal colorectal tumours. Consequently, other *in vivo* models had to be developed for testing the localization of radiolabelled monoclonal antibodies in human tumours.

Tumour xenografts

The method most widely used has been to grow the appropriate human tumours in animals as xenografts. Such xenograft models have also been widely exploited to test chemotherapeutic agents against human tumours in the *in vivo* setting. Foreign tissues, such as human tumours, would not normally grow in animals, of course, because the animal's immune system would recognise the tissue as foreign, mount an immune response against it, and it would be rejected. Growth of such xenografts therefore requires the animals immune system to be evaded or depressed. One way to avoid the immune system is to grow the tumour in a so-called immunologically privileged site, where, mainly for anatomical reasons, the animal's immune mechanisms, particularly the cell-mediated response mainly responsible for tissue rejection, cannot reach. One such widely used site in early studies was the cheek pouch of the hamster. For example, some of the early studies with radioiodine labelled anti-CEA antibodies were carried out with human colon carcinoma grown in this way (Goldenberg et al., 1974). Subsequently techniques were developed to reliably immunosuppress mice so that they could be used to grow a wide range of human tumour types at other anatomical sites. The technique here was to suppress the immune response by removal of the thymus gland from very young animals, followed by whole body irradiation with either subsequent bone marrow reconstitution or treatment just before the irradiation with drugs such as cytosine arabinoside to protect the bone marrow against the effects of irradiation (Steel et al., 1978). A wide range of human tumours were grown in this way, mainly as subcutaneous grafts and were used for testing of chemotherapeutic agents and for examining the localization potential of radiolabelled monoclonal antibodies. For example, in the authors' hands such immunosuppressed mice were used for growth of osteosarcoma and colorectal xenografts used in the pre-clinical evaluation of a number of monoclonal antibodies.

In the mid-1960s a mutation in mice which caused a lack of the thymus was described. These animals had a related genetic defect which caused them to be hairless, and they became officially designated as *nude mice*. The congenital immunological deficiency of these mice is sufficient to allow them to accept xenografts of tissue, including human tumours. These mice are relatively expensive, and because of their immunological incompetence they are prone to infection and so survive and thrive best under barrier conditions. Nevertheless, their increasing commercial availability has led to them superseding artificially immunosuppressed mice or other models for growth of human tumour xenografts in many areas of cancer research, including studies with tumour-localizing monoclonal antibodies.

Although some human tumour types do grow more readily than others, overall all common malignancies against which monoclonal antibodies are available have been reported to have been grown in nude mice. These include particularly colorectal, ovarian, lung, breast, gastric and bladder carcinoma, and melanoma and bone and soft tissue sarcomas. The usual practice is to grow tumours as subcutaneous grafts. Either cells grown in tissue culture can be injected each time, or tissue can be passaged from mouse to mouse, the initial tumour having originated from either human material grown in tissue culture or implanted straight from patient material into the mice. With many human tumour xenograft lines used for experimental imaging with monoclonal antibodies, tumours of one or two centimetre diameters will grow up from small inocula of tissue within a few weeks.

One criticism of the use of subcutaneous tumours in this way is that a tumour of only even a few millimetres in diameter in a mouse weighing only 20 or 30 grams is out of proportion in relation to similar size tumours or metastases in a patient. Furthermore, these subcutaneous tumours in animals are, by virtue of their location, discrete and readily distinguishable from other tissue, favouring their identification by gamma camera imaging. In addition, the antigenic profile, particularly the level of antigen expression and the uniformity of its expression throughout the tumour tissue, may be more favourable than that in tumours in patients. Also their vascularity, rate of blood flow, and indeed their whole architecture may be different from the clinical situation which they are meant to model. These are of course valid criticisms, but nevertheless these xenograft have proved valuable in selecting monoclonal antibodies and their radiolabels for clinical evaluation and understanding the seemingly anomalous differences in the biodistribution and imaging characteristics of labelled antibodies compared with their fragments. Probably most of the monoclonal antibodies which have undergone and which are currently undergoing clinical trials will have been tested for their ability to localize in the appropriate human tumour type grafted to nude mice.

Metastatic tumour xenograft models. In addition to the growth of human tumours as subcutaneous xenografts, a number of techniques to generate disseminated disease with some tumour types have been described. These may be better models of clinical situations. With ovarian cancer, for example (where disease remains largely confined to the peritoneum throughout most of the disease history), intraperitoneal growth of human ovarian cancer in nude mice has been described, including both solid and ascitic growths (Ward et al., 1987) which can be generated by intraperitoneal injection of tumour cells.

To produce tumour growth at other sites, more complex manipulations and surgical procedures may be needed. Thus Mclemore et al., (1987) have described the growth of human lung carcinoma in the lung of nude mice following intrabronchial injection of cells. With colon carcinoma, secondaries in the liver have been produced by initial implantation of cells into the caecal wall of nude mice (Bresalier et al., 1987) or into the spleen from which the cells are drained to the liver (Giavazzi et al., 1986). Some human tumours will produce lymph node secondaries, following, for example, injection into the foot pad of the hind legs (Shah et al., 1987). Sands et al. (1986) have used tumours grown under the renal capsule mice for antibody localization studies. Overall, however, these models have as yet been little used for examining the localization and imaging capacity of monoclonal antibodies, probably because of the technical difficulties involved. The solid subcutaneous tumour model is the most frequently reported for straightforward evaluation of tumour localization potential of antibodies.

Imaging of tumour xenografts. To examine the biodistribution and tumour imaging capacity of radiolabelled monoclonal antibodies in nude mice with human tumour xenografts, it is most appropriate to inject antibody labelled to the same specific antibody as it is envisaged to be used clinically, i.e., in the range of 30–150 MBq/mg. Ideally only a few micrograms of antibody should be injected, so that the dose is more or less equivalent on a body weight basis to that to be used clinically. Radiolabelled antibody given intraperitoneally into experimental animals will rapidly enter the circulation and be available for tumour localization. However, it is usually more appropriate to inject intravenously, via a tail vein, although this is technically more difficult. Gamma camera imaging on such small animals is best carried out with a pin hole collimator with a 2–3 mm diameter inset. Tumour visualization is not usually seen until one or two days after the injection of antibody, although, as will be discussed below, this can depend very much on the radiolabel used and whether intact antibody or fragments are tested.

In addition to imaging, the biodistribution of radiolabelled monoclonal antibody in animals can be assessed by blood sampling and final dissection when radioactivity in organs can be directly measured with a gamma counter. Using this dissection method, the proportion of the injected dose of radiolabel localized per gram of tissue can be calculated. This can be as high as 10–20% of the dose/gram two or three days after injection. Mouse monoclonal antibodies injected into mice have a catabolic half time of usually 2 to 5 days (this depends on the isotype of the antibody but probably varies somewhat from individual antibody to individual antibody). Consequently, when expressed as the proportion of the whole body count rate, tumour localization can be as high as 50%/gram.

In addition to examining the localization of the antibody in question, the xenograft models enable specificity controls to be included in these pre-clinical tests. Thus, as well as testing the antibody in mice with tumours known to be reactive with the antibody, mice with other antigenically negative tumours can also be tested and should show no localisation. In such cases tumour levels of radiolabel should be no higher than those in normal organs such as the liver. Another way of confirming that the tumour localization of radiolabelled antibody is caused by specific antigen recognition is to inject simultaneously antibody with one radiolabel and an unrelated monoclonal antibody or normal immunoglobulin with another. This paired labelling technique with I-131 and I-125 was introduced by Pressman in the 1950s (Pressman et al., 1957) and is still widely used. Iodine-131 and I-125 are convenient labels for this procedure and can be counted simultaneously because of their widely differing energies of gamma emission. Figure 3.1 shows an example of this technique. Nude mice with xenografts of a gastric carcinoma were injected with a mixture of I-131-labelled control IgG2b (isolated from normal mouse serum) and I-125-labelled 791T/36 monoclonal antibody. Mice were killed and dissected after five days and the two radiolabels assayed in weighed samples of tumour and other tissues. There is clear specific localization of the I-125 antibody in tumour tissue, the level of this being about four times that seen with the control IgG2b. Levels of both radiolabels were virtually identical in all of the other, normal, tissues examined. With Indium-111 as the antibody radiolabel it would perhaps be feasible to use Gallium-67 as the radiolabel for control immunoglobulin. These types of specificity tests have now been reported with a wide range of monoclonal antibodies, and have been used to show that there is site-specific antigen-directed localization of many monoclonal antibodies *in vivo*.

Blood pool subtraction techniques for image enhancement. With radioio-

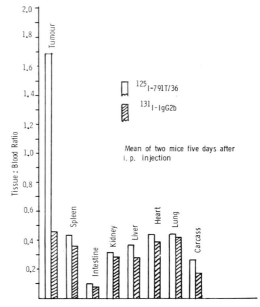

Fig. 3.1. An example from the authors' work of the paired label technique to examine localisation of an monoclonal antibody in subcutaneous xenografts of a human gastric carcinoma in nude mice. I-125-labelled 791T/36 antibody was injected intravenously mixed with I-131-labelled control normal immunoglobulin of the same isotype (IgG2b). Five days later the mice were killed for dissection and the two radiolabels measured simultaneously in weighed samples of tissues. The count rates of the two radiolabels were normalised with respect to those in the blood to give tissue to blood ratios. There is very clear localisation of the antibody in the tumour tissue, the tumour to blood ratio of antibody being four times that of control immunoglobulin. The distributions of the two radiolabels in all other tissues are virtually the same as each other.

dines, particularly I-131, as the radiolabel for monoclonal antibodies rather than radiometals, image quality is not good, this due in part to the relative target, non-target, and blood levels of the different radiolabels. Early on in clinical immunoscintigraphy, when iodine-131 was the most widely used radiolabel, blood pool subtraction methods were advocated for image enhancement. Here a second radiolabel, usually technetium-99m labelled red blood cells or HSA, was given intrave-

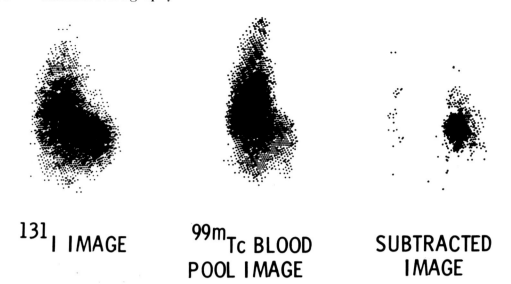

^{131}I IMAGE ^{99m}Tc BLOOD POOL IMAGE   SUBTRACTED IMAGE

Fig. 3.2. An example from the authors' work of a subtraction technique for image enhancement. A mouse with a subcutaneous xenograft of a human colon carcinoma was injected intravenously with I-131-labelled anti-CEA monoclonal antibody. Three days later the distribution of I-131 in the mouse was assessed by imaging with a gamma camera fitted with a pin-hole collimator. Although the tumour can be seen it cannot be clearly delineated from normal tissues. A second image was acquired simultaneously after the intravenous injection of Tc-99m. After normalisation of count rates the blood pool image was subtracted from the antibody distribution image. I-131 localisation in the tumour can now be clearly seen.

nously shortly before imaging to simulate the blood pool. Images of the biodistribution of both the radioiodine and the technetium-99m were acquired, and after count rate normalization, the latter image was subtracted from the former to compensate for radioiodine surviving in the blood to allow more precise tumour discrimination.

The value of this technique was also demonstrated experimentally in nude mice with human tumour xenografts. Figure 3.2 shows an early example from the authors' work. Here nude mice with xenografts of a CEA-producing colon carcinoma had been injected three days before with I-131-labelled anti-CEA monoclonal antibody. The I-131 image showed only poor visualization of the tumour, and a lot of radiolabel is still in the circulation. A blood pool image of the distribution of intravenously injected technetium-99m was acquired si-

multaneously. This, a characteristic blood pool image, showed radiolabel in the liver, heart, etc. There is some activity in the tumour because, of course, the tumour does have a vasculature. But subtraction of the technetium-99m blood pool image from that of the I-131 showed clearly the position of the subcutaneous tumour.

Other refinements in immunoscintigraphy, particularly the use of radiometals, has obviated the need for such image enhancement techniques, but these experimental systems are available for evaluation of other image enhancement methods. For example, other blood pool simulators are available, such as free indium-113m, which will attach to serum transferrin and which has been used in image enhancement methods both experimentally and clinically.

Both technetium-99m and indium-113m image enhancement methods attempt to simulate the distribution of the intravascular blood pool in tumour and normal organs. But a more appropriate method would be to simulate the background biodistribution of the monoclonal antibody since this, because of the intra- and extravascular distribution pattern, will not be precisely simulated by a marker which is predominantly intravascular. One way to do this would be to administer at the same time as the radiolabelled monoclonal antibody normal immunoglobulin or an irrelevant monoclonal antibody labelled with another radionuclide which could be imaged simultaneously with the antibody. This normal immunoglobulin's biodistribution should be virtually identical to that of the monoclonal antibody, except where the latter is deposited specifically in the target lesion. With iodine-131 as the label for the antibody, iodine-123-labelled control immunoglobulin could be used. With radiometals, indium-111 labelled antibody could be paired with gallium-67 labelled control immunoglobulin. The experimental xenografts models available could be used to evaluate these methods, although so far there has been little reported work in this area.

Influence of circulating antigen on antibody biodistribution. It is quite possible that the antigens identified by monoclonal antibodies within tumours can be released into the circulation. This is certainly the case with antigens such as CEA where monitoring circulating levels can be used diagnostically/prognostically. Other antigens may be secreted products like CEA, or they may be released following tumour cell death/necrosis. Whatever the precise source of antigen in the circulation, it could potentially have a detrimental effect on tumour imaging. Circulating antigen, able to form immune complexes with intravenously injected monoclonal antibodies, have certainly been identified in

patients with germ cell tumours, colorectal carcinoma, and ovarian carcinoma. It is possible that the circulating antigen could complex with monoclonal antibody, neutralizing its ability to localize in tumour tissue and possibly resulting in immune complexes being deposited in the liver or spleen with corresponding detrimental effect on images. In most clinical situations this does not in fact seem to occur, and although the formation of immune complexes certainly takes place, these seem to remain in the circulation and image quality is not affected. The survival of these complexes, and unperturbed deposition of antibody in tumours, allowing successful imaging still to be achieved, is rather an unexpected finding, and one for which an experimental model would be of value.

However, mice with the corresponding xenografts of human tumours rarely have circulating tumour-derived antigen. The reason for this is unclear, but it means that there are few xenograft models for investigation of this phenomenon. One exception is the report by Hagan et al., (1985) with a CEA-producing colon carcinoma xenograft and anti-CEA antibody, where it was shown that radiolabelled antibody was cleared, particularly to the liver and spleen, putatively as immune complexes. Mice with tumours producing the highest level of CEA showed the most pronounced clearance. In addition, with the 19.9 anti-colorectal carcinoma monoclonal antibodies, Douilland et al., (1985) found that localization into colon carcinoma xenografts was poor with uptake of antibody radiolabel into liver and spleen. The 19.9 defined antigen was found in the circulation, and it was assumed but not formally shown that immune complexes were formed and cleared. With $F(ab')_2$ fragments of the antibody, there was more effective tumour localization, the interpretation here being that while immune complexes forming

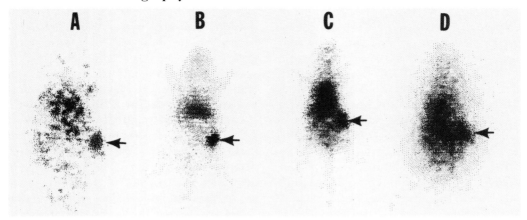

Fig. 3.3. A demonstration from the authors' studies of the effect on tumour imaging of the radionuclide used to label the monoclonal antibody. Here mice with subcutaneous xenografts of a human osteogenic sarcoma were injected with 791T/36 labelled monoclonal antibody labelled with Tc-99m(A), In-111(B), I-123(C), or I-131(D). Compared with I-131, the physical characteristics of I-123 result in clearer tumour imaging. However even better images of tumours were achieved with In-111- or Tc-99m-labelled antibody, and this cannot be due only to differences in their energies of gamma emission.

with intact antibody could be cleared into liver and spleen (probably by recognition of the Fc portion of the complex), those with fragments (lacking the Fc) could not and so tumour localization was still possible.

It has not been explained why it is that in those few xenograft systems where circulating antigen can be identified perturbed biodistribution of radiolabelled monoclonal antibody is observed while such perturbation does not seem to be a problem clinically. It may be that complexes formed between mouse monoclonal antibody and antigen are cleared more readily by the reticuloendothelial system of mouse than they are by man's. Immune complexes between mouse monoclonal antibody and anti-mouse antibody generated by patients are cleared from the circulation, but this could be due to easier recognition in man of immune complexes containing human antibody. These problems of the effects of circulating antigen on tumour imaging still require adequate experimental models for their investigation.

Biodistribution and imaging characteristics of antibodies radiolabelled with different radionuclides. The different radionuclides used for labelling antibodies for immunoscintigraphy have different physical characteristics, and their different energies of gamma emission will clearly influence the relative efficiencies of photon detection and of collimation and scatter characteristics, all of which will affect image quality. At first sight, leaving aside differences in half-lives, it would be expected that image quality obtained with any one antibody labelled with the four most commonly used radiolabels for immunoscintigraphy, that is iodine-123, iodine-131, indium-111, and technetium-99m, would be ranked in the order of their gamma energies. It would be expected that technetium-99m (141 keV) would be the best, followed by iodine-123 (159 keV), indium-111 (173 and 247 keV), and iodine 131 (364 keV). In practice this is not the case, and tumour xenograft models have been of great value in understanding the relative imaging efficiencies of

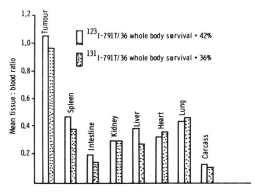

Fig. 3.4. An experimental comparison of the biodistribution and tumour localisation of I-123- and I-131-labelled monoclonal antibody. Mice with xenografts of human osteogenic sarcoma were injected separately with labelled 791T/36 antibody. Images of the mice injected with I-123-labelled material showed clearer tumour identification (see Fig. 3.3). This was probably due to the different energies of gamma emission of the two radioiodines. It would not be expected that there would be any difference in the *biological* behaviour of the two preparations, and this was confirmed when the mice were dissected after three days. An example from the authors' studies.

these different radiolabels. They will no doubt be of value in studying the relative biodistributions and imaging characteristics of newer radiolabels such as gallium-67 and lead-203, which are being considered, as well as the different characteristics of an antibody labelled with any one radionuclide by different methods of conjugation.

The different imaging characteristics of a particular antibody with different radiolabels can be illustrated here by some of the authors' work on comparing the imaging of human osteosarcoma xenografts in immunodeprived mice. Here tumours were transplanted subcutaneously, and the imaging characteristics assessed using a monoclonal antibody labelled with the four radionuclides were compared (Fig. 3.3). All the images were acquired 3 days after injection of the radiolabelled monoclonal antibody. The images obtained with iodine-131-labelled antibody were poor,

with a large amount of scatter, high blood pool activity, and no really clear-cut discrimination of the tumour site. The images with iodine-123 had much less scatter, and the tumour sites could be distinguished. However, with indium-111, whose energies of gamma emission are higher than iodine-123, tumour discrimination was vastly improved! Images with technetium-99m were technically poor because these were acquired two days after injection and there was little remaining activity, but tumour discrimination was good and more comparable with those seen with indium-111.

Since all the radiolabelled preparations were of the same antibody (and all of equal purity and immunological reactivity), the finding of the imaging studies are at first sight paradoxical. Why does the image quality not correlate with the energies of gamma emission of the radionuclides? As we will see later in Chapter 4, this volume, dealing with clinical imaging, this is not a peculiarity of the experimental animal system, and the clinical results bear out the experimental finding. The reason is only explained by data from the animal studies and is related to the different physiological fates of the radiolabels after catabolism of the antibody.

With the antibody labelled with iodine-123 and iodine-131, dissection of the mice and assay of the radioiodines in samples of blood, tumour, and other tissues shows the biodistributions to be virtually identical (Fig. 3.4). This is as would be expected, since the radiolabelled antibody was of equal quality in both cases, and iodine-123 and iodine-131 obviously cannot be distinguished between physiologically. Thus it can only be concluded that the differences in the images are due to the different characteristics of gamma emission.

In contrast, dissection analysis of mice injected with iodine-131- or indium-111-

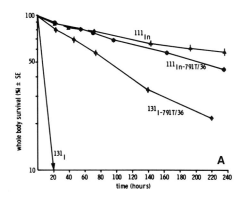

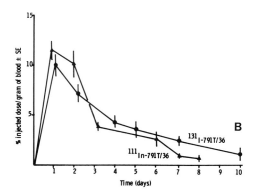

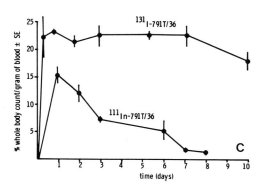

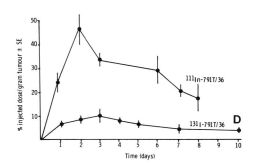

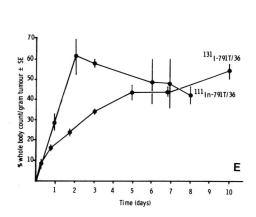

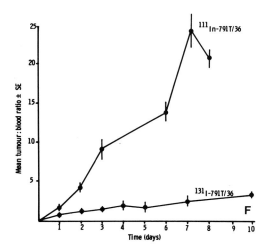

labelled antibody showed quite different biodistributions of the two radiolabels. The whole body retention of indium-111 following injection of labelled antibody was significantly longer than that of iodine-131 following injection of iodine-131-labelled antibody (Fig. 3.5A), with biological retention half times of 200 hours and 90 hours, respectively. However, the blood levels of the two radiolabels and the rates of their clearance were virtually identical (Fig. 3.5B). Free iodine-131, given as sodium iodide, was excreted rapidly, as would be expected, since unless incorporated into thyroxine in the thyroid, iodine is rapidly excreted in the urine, with a little uptake in the salivary glands and the gastric mucosa. Free indium-111, given as indium chloride, was lost much more slowly. This also is to be expected, since it is known indium can become attached to serum proteins such as transferrin in the same way as can iron, and is subsequently removed from the blood and retained, in some way, in virtually all tissues of the body. Eventually it is excreted, but only slowly, in both faeces and urine. Thus it is

likely that the differences in whole body retention of the two radiolabels on the antibody is a reflection of the rates of excretion of these radionuclides following antibody catabolism rather than a reflection of different rates of catabolism of the two labelled antibody preparations. The indication is that when radioiodine is freed from antibody, it is excreted rapidly from the body, probably as free iodine or as iodotyrosine, whereas when radioindium is released, it is retained at the site of catabolism.

One consequence of this is that, although the absolute blood levels of radioiodine and radioindium labelled preparations are the same, the levels in relation to the whole body count rate are quite different, those of radioiodine being maintained at much higher levels (Fig. 3.5C). Consequently, because gamma cameras scale the levels of radioactivity relative to that in the most radioactive region, imaging would be expected to show an apparent clearance of radioindium from the blood pool, since radioactivity is progressively associated with other normal tissues

Fig. 3.5. An experimental examination of the different biological behaviour of radioindium and radioiodine after injection of labelled monoclonal antibody. Mice were injected intraperitoneally with free radioiodide, free radioindium or monoclonal antibody 791T/36 labelled with either of the two radionuclides. A: Survival of radiolabels in the whole body. Free radioiodide was rapidly excreted and the loss of radioiodine after injection of labelled antibody is therefore a measure of the rate of catabolism of the antibody. However free radioindium was excreted only slowly and it is therefore unlikely that the rate of excretion of radioindium from labelled antibody can be taken as a measure of the rate of catabolism of the antibody. B: A comparison of blood levels of radiolabels expressed as the proportion of the dose/gram of blood. Blood levels of the two radiolabels were virtually identical over a ten day period indicating similar blood survival of the antibody with either label. Contrast this with the whole body retention of the radiolabels seen in panel A. C: A comparison of blood levels of radiolabels expressed as a proportion of the count rate surviving in the whole animal. Blood levels of radioindium are lower than those of radioiodine when expressed in this way. Thus imaging of tumours with radioindium labelled antibody would be favoured by the relatively low normal tissue to blood ratio. D: A comparison of tumour xenograft levels of radiolabels. Tumour retains a higher proportion of the injected dose of radioindium/gram of tissue. This also would favour tumour imaging with radioindium. E: A comparison of tumour levels of the two radiolabels expressed as a proportion of the total count rate surviving in the animal. Although the prolonged retention of radioindium (panel A) could tend to reduce tumour to normal tissue ratios the even greater retention in tumour means that tumour to normal tissues ratios are higher than those seen with radioiodine. F: A comparison of tumour levels of the two radiolabels expressed as a tumour to blood ratio. The levels of radioindium in the tumour are higher than those of radioiodine (panel D), but blood levels are the same (panel B). Consequently tumour to blood ratios are higher with radioindium than with radioiodine. (Reproduced from Pimm et al., Eur. J. Nucl. Med. 11:300–304, 1985, with permission of the publisher.)

within the field of view. Organ distribution studies in mice show that it is particularly spleen, liver, and kidney that retain the radioindium, while heart and lung show higher levels of radioiodine. Retention of tracer within the liver is a consistent finding with all indium-labelled antibodies in both experimental and clinical studies. Tumour tissue shows a two-to-three-fold increase in the proportion of the dose of radioindium per gram of tissue compared with radioiodine (Fig. 3.5D), suggesting that tumour tissue also has the propensity to retain the radiometal after its delivery via antibody. Expressed as the proportion of the count rate in the whole body field of view, tumour levels are higher with indium-111 labelled antibody than with iodine-131 for at least five or six days after injection (Fig. 3.5E). Expressed as tumour to blood ratios, this difference is even more striking (Fig. 3.5F).

Overall, this and similar imaging and related dissection studies in experimental systems (Khaw et al., 1986; Brown et al., 1987) have helped to explain the superior imaging characteristics seen with radioindium-labelled antibodies in clinical trials. The conclusion is that superior imaging with radioindium compared with radioiodines is due to a fortuitous combination of circumstances. Certainly the lower energy of gamma emission with indium-111 facilitates its detection, but retention in normal tissues such as liver and bone marrow of indium released during antibody catabolism produces a relative blood pool clearance of indium compared with iodine, and this facilitates target imaging particularly in vascular regions. In addition, certainly with tumours, the target tissue retains indium more efficiently than it does iodine, and this increases target to non-target ratios, which adds to the superior imaging characteristics.

There seem to be few reported studies on a comparison of the biodistribution of antibodies labelled with radioiodine and with technetium-99m to ascertain whether the superior imaging, which can no doubt be achieved with the technetium labelled preparations, is due to the advantageous physical characteristics or whether relative differences in the metabolic fate of the two radiolabels can contribute to this in the way in which it does with indium labelled antibodies. What evidence there is is equivocal, but suggests that the radiolabel from radioiodine and radiotechnetium labelled proteins tend to behave similarly. The relative distribution and catabolic fate of technetium could, however, depend on the method of linkage to the antibody and, as we saw in Chapter 2, this volume, techniques for optimum labelling are still being developed. Animal models will be useful in determining the target-localizing capacity of these differently labelled preparations and in understanding the distribution seen on imaging.

The intra-tissue catabolism of monoclonal antibodies and their radiolabels, which can affect the relative imaging capabilities of antibodies with different radiolabels, is as yet poorly understood, but is obviously important because it is the continued retention of the radiolabelled antibody, or at least of the radiolabel as it accumulates in the target tissue, which produces the discrimination between target and non-target tissues. Overall the available evidence suggests that radioindium and radioiodine labelled antibodies distribute and behave similarly, but while the iodine is excreted following catabolism in the tissues, the radioindium is retained, although really neither the mechanism of antibody catabolism nor the mechanism of retention of the radioindium is understood as yet (Sands and Jones, 1987). It is not really known whether antibody is catabolized differently in, say tumour tissue, than it is in corresponding normal tissues. Certainly antibody is metabolized following immune fixation in tumour, as has been shown by the identification of antibody breakdown products in experimental tumours such as human tumour xenografts in athymic mice (Endo et al., 1987). It is known that the whole body catabolic rate of radioiodine labelled antibodies is increased in animals with tumours showing localization of that antibody (Pimm and Baldwin, 1987), but the intra-tissue fate of radioindium under these circumstances is unclear.

It has been suggested that the ubiquitous tissue retention of indium is due to binding to polyanionic mucopolysaccharides in connective tissue, or it could be retained on iron-binding proteins (Wochner et al., 1970; Dassin et al., 1978; Fowler et al., 1983). Whatever the mechanism, this is an important characteristic of radioindium labelled antibodies which requires further study, almost certainly requiring the use of animal models. In parallel, it is equally important to understand the liver retention of radioindium from labelled antibodies because this is one of the major disadvantages of this particular radiolabel compared with radioiodine for imaging abdominal tumours and, of course, for the detection of liver metastasis. The available evidence suggests that this too is due more to prolonged retention of the radioindium in the liver than to any fundamental difference in the biodistribution of antibody with the different radiolabels. It is to be expected that the development of different methods of linking radioindium to antibodies, with different chelators and maybe site-specific labelling (see Chapter 2, this volume), will perhaps overcome this problem of liver retention of the radioindium, and it can be envisaged

that experimental models will play a major part in the evaluation of those preparations.

Biodistribution and imaging characteristics of antibody fragments. Fragments of IgG antibodies, particularly $F(ab')_2$ and Fab, produced by enzyme digestion of antibodies, have been known for many years to have quite different biodistribution characteristics and rates of biological degradation than their parent antibodies. In early studies of the biodistribution of antibodies these and other defined fragments were useful in determining the biological role of different parts of the immunoglobulin molecule. For example, it is usually thought now that the Fc part of the immunoglobulin molecule is in some way involved in controlling its rate of catabolism. In mice, for example, intact antibodies have biological half-times of several days, depending on the particular isotype of the immunoglobulin, while fragments, lacking the Fc portion, have a biological half-life measured more in hours than in days. The smaller molecular size of fragments allows more rapid diffusion from the blood into extravascular spaces and a higher proportion of the fragments is resident extravascularly, in the interstitial spaces of the tissues (Covell et al., 1986).

Some of these characteristics of antibody fragments and their bearing on their application to immunoscintigraphy can be illustrated here by some of the authors' work. Thus in studies with a mouse monoclonal antibody, against CEA, the intact IgG antibody, after intravenous injection into normal mice, was cleared initially from the blood (α phase) with a half-time of 9.9 hours, representing mainly the distribution of the antibody between the intra- and extravascular compartments (Fig. 3.6A). Subsequently, after about 24 hours, blood clearance was much slower, with a

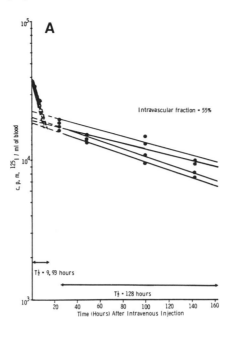

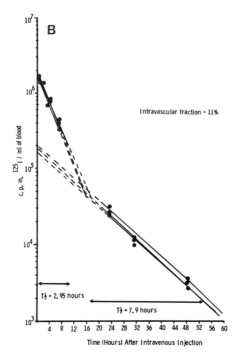

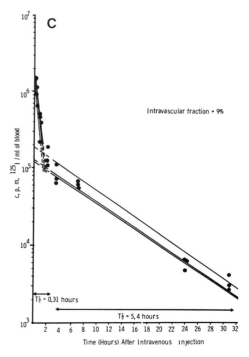

half time of 128 hours, this β phase representing the rate of overall catabolism of the antibody. Using methods worked out many years previously in the study of the distribution and catabolism of serum proteins, it is possible to extrapolate the β phase to the y axis to give the hypothetical blood count rate at time zero assuming that extravasation had taken place but that no antibody has been lost by catabolism. By relating this to the actual blood level immediately after injection, the proportion of antibody going into the intra- and extravascular compartments can be calculated. With this antibody the intravascular retention was calculated to be 55%. In sharp contrast, the $F(ab')_2$ fragment of this antibody had a α phase half-time of 2.9 hours, a β phase of 7.9 hours, and an intravascular fraction of only 11% (Fig. 3.6B). The Fab fragment was catabolized even more rapidly, with an α phase half-time of only 0.3 hours and a β of 5.4 hours, with an intravascular fraction of 9% (Fig. 3.6C). These and similar studies with monoclonal antibody fragments suggested that tumour localization of fragments may be more efficient than that of intact antibody.

Because fragments extravasate more rapidly, and to a higher degree, earlier and/or greater tumour deposition of antibody should be possible, since obviously this depends on the antibody extravasating to reach target antigen. Other factors influencing the possible tumour imaging efficiency of fragments compared with intact antibody have become clear from animal model studies and have been useful in predicting and explaining clinical findings. Fragments, particularly Fab, are small enough to be cleared into the kidney, and available evidence suggests that they are actually catabolized there. With radioiodine labelled fragments, therefore, high kidney levels of tracer can be seen, often within a few hours of injection. The more rapid overall catabolism and excretion of radioiodine labelled fragments also results in radioactivity appearing in the urinary tract. Accumulation of radioiodine may also occur in the stomach due to secretion at this site.

The overall increase in the rate of catabolism of antibody fragments means that, while they may localize faster in tumour sites, the absolute proportion in tumour tissue is greatly reduced and the count rate available for imaging will also be reduced. This can be illustrated with distribution studies in nude mice, with CEA-producing xenografts injected with fragments of the same anti-CEA antibody referred to above. Kinetic studies with intact antibody showed peak tumour levels 24 hours after injection, at 20% of the dose/gram of tumour tissue, this being higher than normal organs, including liver, kidneys, and stomach, and also higher than that of blood (Fig. 3.7A). With the $F(ab)_2$ fragments, kidney and stomach had the highest initial

---

Fig. 3.6. A comparison in experimental animals of the relative blood clearance and catabolism of intact anti-CEA antibody and its $F(ab)_2$ and Fab fragments. Mice were injected intravenously with radioiodine labelled preparations and blood samples taken for radioactivity counting. A: Intact antibody. Radiolabel leaves the blood with an initial (α) extravasation half-time of 9.9 hours, followed by a catabolic (β) phase with a 128-hour half-time. Extrapolation of the β phase back to the ordinate shows that after the extravasation phase the remaining antibody has distributed so that 55% is intravascular, and 45% extravascular. B: $F(ab)_2$. Both the α and β phases have much shorter half-times than those of intact antibody. The intravascular fraction is now only 11%. Thus the fragment moves more quickly and to a greater extent out of the blood into the tissues, but also undergoes far more rapid catabolism. C: Fab. Both α and β phases have half-times even shorter than those of $F(ab)_2$. Overall it could be expected that fragments would show greater and more rapid tumour discrimination than intact antibody. (From the authors' unpublished studies.)

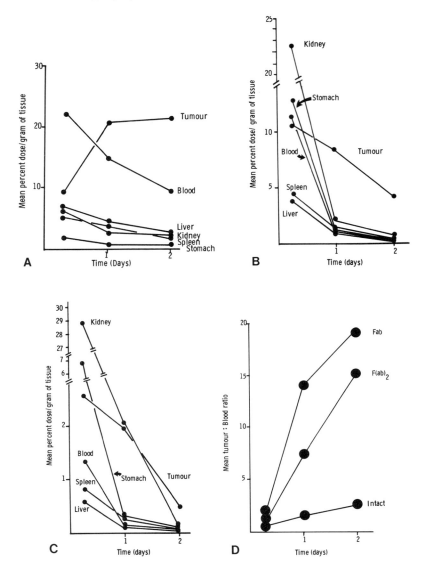

Fig. 3.7. A comparison of tumour and normal tissue levels of radiolabelled intact anti-CEA antibody and its F(ab)$_2$ and Fab fragments. Mice with subcutaneous xenografts of a human gastric carcinoma were injected intravenously with radioiodine labelled preparations and dissected at three different time points. **A:** Intact antibody takes 24 hours to reach peak tumour levels, but by this time each gram of tumour has 20% of the dose. **B:** F(ab)$_2$ has reached peak levels in the tumour by 6 hours, but this is only 10% of the dose/gram and there are higher levels in kidney, stomach, and blood. Tumour levels then decline, but not as rapidly as those in normal tissues. **C:** Fab reaches peak levels in tumour by 6 hours, but at only 3%/gram, not as high as levels in kidney and stomach. High kidney levels were present throughout the time course studied. **D:** A comparison of tumour discrimination with antibody and fragments, expressed here as a tumour to blood ratio. Fab and F(ab)$_2$ give much higher ratios, although this has been achieved at the expense of much lower absolute levels of fragment localising in tumour tissue (see panels A–C). (Reproduced from Pimm et al., Nucl. Med. Commun. 10:585–593, 1989, with permission from the publisher.)

levels of radiolabel, and although they had fallen by 24 hours after injection to less than that of tumour, the levels in tumour were at maximum 11% of the dose/gram, and this declined over the next two days. Blood levels of radiolabel were, after one day, much lower than those in tumour (Fig. 3.7B). With Fab fragments, kidney and stomach levels of radioiodine were even higher, tumour levels of radiolabel were at best only 2.5% of the dose/gram, and were no higher than those of the kidney until at least two days after injection (Fig. 3.7C).

These different catabolic and biodistribution characteristics produced quite different degrees of tumour discrimination. Intact antibody gave the highest absolute amount in tumour tissue, but the lowest tumour to blood ratios, while Fab gave the lowest absolute levels in tumour but the highest tumour to blood ratio, this being about 6 times that of intact antibody (Fig. 3.7D). These dissection analyses help to explain the images of such xenografted mice injected with I-131-labelled antibody and fragments (Andrew et al., 1988). Thus tumour is seen with intact antibody with any confidence only by three days (Fig. 3.8A). With F(ab)₂, tumour could be seen by 6 hours, and at 72 hours the images were far superior to those with the intact antibody (Fig. 3.8B). With Fab, although tumour could be seen at 6 hours, kidney and particularly bladder activity dominated the images. By 72 hours, tumour was very clearly seen, although the overall low count rate was now a limitation (Fig. 3.8C).

As we saw above, the radiolabel used for a monoclonal antibody can, both for physical and biological reasons, have a great influence on its tumour imaging capability. Because radiometals, particularly Indium-111, have such superior properties with antibodies, and fragments have such superior properties over intact antibody, it was

tempting to speculate that Indium-111 labelled fragments would have ever greater imaging efficiency. Studies in mice with xenografts have shown, however, that the situation is not as clear as it was hoped (Andrew et al., 1988; Brown et al., 1987). Because fragments are catabolized so quickly, and radioindium tends to be retained at the site of catabolism rather than being excreted like radioiodine, these sites of catabolism, particularly the kidneys, tend to dominate images of mice with xenografts given Indium-111 labelled fragments, especially Fab (Fig. 3.8C). Although tumour localization does occur, imaging with fragments, at least with Fab, is more clear-cut with radioiodine than with radioindium. These findings with xenograft models are, as discussed later, relevant to understanding the different imaging characteristics of antibodies and fragments with different radiolabels.

Human monoclonal antibodies. Human monoclonal antibodies are currently being developed as an alternative to mouse antibodies, particularly against human tumour associated antigens (Chapter 1, this volume). Currently these are undergoing preclinical evaluation for immunoscintigraphy in nude mice with appropriate human tumour xenografts. Many of these antibodies are IgMs, unlike the mouse monoclonal antibodies where predominantly IgGs are produced. Thus it is clear that a future area of investigation in animal systems will be the biodistribution and tumour localization potential of IgM antibodies.

IgM antibodies have a biodistribution different from that of IgG antibodies. They generally have a shorter biological half-life than IgG antibodies, of the order of a half to one day for mouse IgMs in mice, and a greater intravascular fraction due to their larger size. Nevertheless, they have been shown to localize in experimental tumours

A

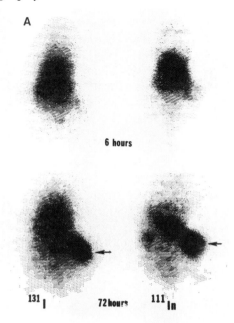

6 hours

^{131}I   72 hours ^{111}In

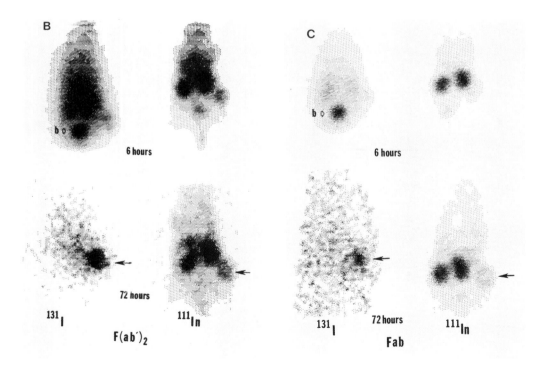

B   6 hours   C   6 hours

b ◊   b ◊

72 hours   72 hours

^{131}I ^{111}In ^{131}I ^{111}In

F(ab´)$_2$ Fab

(Ballou et al., 1985; Maillet et al., 1985). Fragments of mouse IgM antibodies, particularly monomeric forms produced by breakdown of the IgM pentamer and F(ab')$_2$ fragments, termed F(ab')$_2\mu$, can be produced, and have been compared with intact IgM antibodies for tumour localization in mouse tumour systems. The half times of the fragments of IgM antibodies are much more similar to that of the parent antibody than are fragments of the IgG antibodies.

The only report to date with human IgM monoclonal antibodies is that of McCabe et al., (1988), who have demonstrated that following radioiodination two human IgM monoclonal antibodies against human colon carcinoma localized in and could be used for imaging colon carcinoma xenografts in nude mice.

Limitations of tumour xenografts.
Although nude mice with human tumour xenografts have proved valuable in selecting monoclonal antibodies with clinical imaging potential, there are two major criticisms of nude mice xenografts as clinical models which cannot be ignored, and other models are perhaps needed for experimental examination.

The first is that the only human tissue growing in the nude mice is the human tumour. It is unlikely that the majority of monoclonal antibodies against tumour-associated antigens are truly tumour-specific, and it is more likely that the antigens they identify are expressed on some normal tissues, albeit at lower levels than on tumour cells. In the clinical situation, therefore, antibody may react with some normal tissues at low level in addition to the tumour. This may cause some difficulty in image interpretation, and might also have some bearing on the finding that, in clinical imaging, sensitivity sometimes increases with antibody dose. This phenomenon may be due to a considerable proportion of a low dose of antibody being absorbed by normal tissue, whereas a higher dose can saturate low-level antigen expression on normal tissue, leaving adequate antibody available for higher uptake in tumour sites. Obviously the nude mouse model would not be expected to show this phenomenon, and the proposed explanation of dose-dependent clinical imaging is hard to evaluate experimentally with monoclonal antibodies against human tumour-associated antigens. There is some evidence from studies with mouse monoclonal antibodies against animal tumours that this phenomenon may indeed occur. Thus in studies with a monoclonal antibody putatively specific for a mammary carcinoma in rats, the present authors have shown dose-dependent pharmacokinetics and tumour discrimination (Pimm et al., 1986). In this study using a rat model system, blood survival increased as the ad-

Fig. 3.8. The use of a tumour xenograft model for a comparison of the tumour imaging potential of I-131- and In-111-labelled intact anti-CEA antibody and its F(ab)$_2$ and Fab fragments. Mice with subcutaneous xenografts of a human gastric carcinoma were injected intravenously with the preparations and gamma camera imaged at 6 and 72 hours. A: With intact antibody, tumour can be seen only at 72 hours with either I-131 or In-111, although In-111 gives better tumour discrimination in spite of high liver levels of the radiolabel. B: With F(ab)$_2$, tumour can be seen at 6 hours. Excretion of I-131 is seen as radiolabel in the bladder (b). By 72 hours tumour can be very clearly seen with I-131-labelled fragment, but with radioindium kidneys dominate the view. C: With Fab, tumour cannot be seen at 6 hours, the views being dominated by radioactivity in the bladder in the case of I-131 and the kidneys with In-111. By 72 hours, I-131 labelled fragment clearly distinguishes the tumour, but with In-111-labelled fragment the radiolabel has been retained in the kidneys and these still dominate the image. (Reproduced from Andrew et al., Eur. J. Nucl. Med. 13:598–604, 1988, with permission from the publisher.)

ministered protein dose increased, and while low doses of antibody showed accumulation in lung, kidney, and intestine as well as subcutaneous tumour grafts, this was not seen with higher doses, and tumour discrimination was therefore increased (Pimm et al., 1986). Similar dose-dependent biodistribution was seen in rats without tumour, and the probable explanation here is that some normal tissues reacted with the antibody. Subsequent immunohistology revealed definite reaction with intestine and possible reaction with lung and kidney.

The second criticism of the nude mice xenograft model is that these animals, receiving monoclonal antibody for imaging, cannot produce an antibody reaction to the monoclonal antibody, whereas, as shown in Chapter 6, this volume, this is a major problem in repeated injection of monoclonal antibodies to patients. With mouse monoclonal antibodies, mice would not be expected to produce a marked reaction because the monoclonal antibody is of the same species and only anti-idiotypic response might be evoked. But even if antibodies of other species were injected, nude mice would be unable to produce an immune response because of their immunodepressed state, which is necessary in the first instance to allow the human tumour to grow. As discussed in Chapter 6, this volume, immunocompetent animals such as rats or rabbits have been used to examine the immune responses evoked against mouse monoclonal antibodies, and these responses can alter the biodistribution of radiolabelled antibodies. These systems cannot be used, however, to examine the effect of these responses on tumour-imaging capacity of labelled antibodies. This would require tumours grown in immunocompetent animals and monoclonal antibody to be from a different species from that in which the tumour is growing.

Although mouse monoclonal antibodies have been made to antigens associated with tumours in other animal species, such as rat or guinea pig, and used for imaging, the production and biological effects of antibody responses to these mouse antibodies has not been studied.

OTHER PATHOLOGICAL CONDITIONS

Although tumours have attracted the most interest as targets for immunoscintigraphy, monoclonal antibodies suitable for use in several other pathological lesions are now becoming available and model systems are being developed for their pre-clinical evaluation.

Myocardial Infarction

Irreversible ischaemic tissue injury results in the loss of cell membrane integrity. Thus antibody against an otherwise normal intracellular antigen could be localized *in vivo* at the site of tissue injury, either because there has been local leakage of intracellular material, or because antibody, otherwise excluded by the membrane of viable cells, can now penetrate intracellularly. This is the basis of the proposed use of monoclonal antibodies against cardiac myosin in the imaging of myocardial infarction. Animal model systems have contributed to the development of these antibodies from early on. Thus one of the earliest uses of indium-111 labelled antibodies in imaging pathological lesions was the use of anti-myosin in experimentally induced myocardial infarction in dogs (Khaw et al., 1980). Infarction can be induced by ligation of the left anterior descending coronary artery for several hours. The early experimental studies showed imaging twenty-four to forth-eight hours after intravenous injection of indium-111 labelled antibody. This sort of model system can obviously be exploited to compare the imaging efficiencies of different antibodies, fragments, and different radiolabels, etc., such as has already been carried out in imaging of experimental tumours.

Thrombus Imaging With Anti-Fibrin and Anti-Platelet Monoclonal Antibodies

Radiolabelled antibodies were examined in the past as specific probes for thrombi. Antibodies reactive with fibrinogen were used. These became attached to circulating fibrinogen and traced its incorporation into forming thrombi. More recently monoclonal antibodies against fibrin, which react with parts of the molecule not exposed in fibrinogen, have been produced and offer the possibility of imaging thrombi more directly. Experimental imaging of thrombi in animal models has been described, particularly with $F(ab')_2$ and Fab fragments labelled with indium-111. Two techniques for thrombus formation have been used here. In rabbits the injection of iron particles into the ear, followed by collection of the particles in the jugular vein caused by holding a magnet on the neck of the animal, has been described to induce thrombus formation (Knight et al., 1988). In dogs venous thrombi have been induced in the femoral vein by transcatheter placement of embolization coils (Knight et al., 1988; Rosebrough et al., 1988). Both fresh and aged thrombi could be imaged in these model systems within 4 to 24 hours after administration of the antibody, and thrombus localization of the antibody or fragments was confirmed by assay of radiolabels in thrombi.

Experimental thrombi in dogs have also been used to examine the imaging potential of labelled monoclonal antibodies against platelets, where antibody has been produced, which reacts with both canine and human platelets. Thrombi in dogs could be imaged within two to three hours in peripheral veins and arteries, pulmonary arteries, and the right ventricle (Som et al., 1986). The conclusion from these experimental studies was that such antibodies may be useful for imaging thrombi in man.

Imaging Sites of Infection

Monoclonal antibodies have been produced to a wide range of microorganisms. Their possible use in imaging localized infection has been recently investigated (Rubin et al., 1988). Deep thigh infections with *Pseudomonas aeruginosa* were induced by direct injection. A mouse monoclonal antibody against *P. aeruginosa* Immunotpye I lipopolysaccharide was used, and control studies were carried out with an unrelated monoclonal antibody. Accumulation of both specific and non-specific antibody at the site of infection was seen, but this was greater and more prolonged with the specific monoclonal antibody. These authors concluded form this experimental study that specific monoclonal antibody imaging of localized infection is possible and should be clinically useful.

Imaging Inflammatory Lesions

Imaging of inflammatory lesions with *in vivo* labelled and re-infused polymorphonuclear cells is an established nuclear medicine technique. The generation of monoclonal antibodies against antigens associated with such cells opens up the possibility of direct imaging of inflammatory sites following injection of radiolabelled antibody.

Inflammatory lesions can be induced in animals by local injection of oily emulsions such as Freunds Adjuvant. These lesions, induced in mice, have been used by Collet et al., (1988) to investigate immunoscintigraphy with a monoclonal antibody against a macrophage and polymorphonuclear cell antigen. This model showed that it was possible to obtain scintigraphic images of inflammation with antibody over and above those seen with an unrelated control antibody. The same monoclonal antibody was also able to image transplanted tumours in mice, this being mediated by reaction of the antibody with inflammatory cells within tumour lesions.

REFERENCES AND FURTHER READING

Andrew, S.M., Perkins, A.,C., Pimm, M.V., Baldwin, R.W. (1988): A comparison of iodine and indium labelled anti-CEA intact antibody, F(ab)$_2$ and Fab fragments by imaging tumour xenografts. Eur. J. Nucl. Med. 13:598–604.

Ballou, B., Reiland, J., Levine, G., Knowles, B., Hakala, T.R. (1985): Tumor localization using F(ab′)$_2\mu$ from a monoclonal IgM antibody: Pharmacokinetics. J. Nucl. Med. 26:283–292.

Bresalier, R.S., Raper, S.E., Hujanen, E.S., Kim, Y.S. (1987): A new animal model for human colon cancer metastasis. Int. J. Cancer 39:615–630.

Brown, B.A., Comeau, R.D., Jones, P.I., Liberatore, F.A., Neacy, W.P., Sands, H., Gallagher, B.M. (1987): Pharmacokinetics of the monoclonal antibody B72.3 and its fragments labeled with either iodine-125 or indium-111. Cancer Res. 47: 1149–1154.

Collet, B., Pellen, P., Martin, A., Moisan, A., Bourel, D., Toujas, L. (1988): Scintigraphic detection in mice of inflammatory lesions and tumours by an indium labelled monoclonal antibody directed against Mac-1 antigen. Cancer Immunol. Immunother. 26:237–242.

Covell, D.G., Barbet, J., Holton, O.D., Black, C.D.V., Parker, R.J., Weinstein, J.N. (1986): Pharmacokinetics of monoclonal immunoglobulin G1, F(ab′)$_2$ and Fab′ in mice. Cancer Res. 46:3969–3978.

Dassin, E., Eberlin, A., Briere, J., Dosne, A.M., Najean, Y. (1978): Metabolic fate of indium-111 in the rat. Int. J. Nucl. Med. Biol. 5:34–37.

Dassin, E., Malet, F. (1969): Metabolic fate of indium-111 in the rat. Int. J. Nucl. Med. Biol. 5:34–37.

Douillard, J.Y., Chatal, J.F., Curtet, C., Kremer, M., Peuvrel, P., Koprowski, H. (1985): Pharmacokinetic study of radiolabeled anti-colo-rectal carcinoma monoclonal antibodies in tumor-bearing nude mice. Eur. J. Nucl. Med. 11:107–113.

Endo, L., Kamma, H., Ogato, T. (1987): Radiolocalization of xenografted human lung cancer with monoclonal antibody 8 in nude mice. Cancer Res. 47:5427–5432.

Fowler, B.A., Kardish, R.M., Woods, J.S. (1983): Alteration of hepatic microsomal structure and function by indium chloride. Lab Invest. 48:471–477.

Giavazzi, R., Jessup, J.M., Campbell, D.E., Walker, S.M., Fidler, I. (1986): Experimental nude mouse model of human colorectal cancer liver metastases. J. Natl. Cancer Inst. 77:1303–1308.

Goldenberg, D.M., Preston, D.F., Primus, F.J., Hansen, H.J. (1974): Photoscan localization of GW-39 tumors in hamsters using radiolabeled anti-carcinoembryonic antigen immunoglobulin G. Cancer Res. 34:1–9.

Hagan, P.L., Halpern, S.E., Chen, A., Krisnan, L., Frincke, J., Bartholomew, R.M., David, G.S., Carlo, D. (1985): In vivo kinetics of radiolabeled monoclonal anti-CEA antibodies in animal models. J. Nucl. Med. 26:1418–1423.

Khaw, B.A., Fallon, J.T., Strauss, H.W., Haber, E. (1980): Myocardial infarct imaging of antibodies to canine cardiac myosin with indium-111-diethylenetriamine pentaacetic acid. Science 209: 295–297.

Khaw, B.A., Cooney, J., Edgington, T., Strauss, H.W. (1986): Differences in experimental tumour localization of dual labeled monoclonal antibody. J. Nucl. Med. 27:1293–1299.

Knight, L.C., Maurer, A.H., Ammar, I.A., Shealy, D.J., Mattis, J.A. (1988): Evaluation of indium-111-labeled anti-fibrin antibody for imaging vascular thrombi. J. Nucl. Med. 29:494–502.

Maillet, T., Roche, A.C., Therain, F., Mosigney, M. (1985): Time course localization of immunoglobulin M monoclonal antibody and its fragments in leukemic tumor-bearing mice. Cancer Immunol. Immunother. 19:177–182.

McCabe, R.P., Peters, L.C., Haspel, M.V., Pomato, N., Carrasquillo, J.A., Hanna, M.G. (1988): Preclinical studies on the pharmacokinetic properties of human monoclonal antibodies to colo-rectal cancer and their use for detection of tumors. Cancer Res. 48:4348–4353.

Mclemore, T.L., Liu, M.C., Blacker, P.C., Gregg, M., Alley, M.C., Abbott, B.J., Shoemaker, R.H., Bohlman, M.E., Litterst, C.C., Hubbard, W.C., Brennan, R.H., McMahon, J.B., Fine, D.L., Eggleston, J.C., Mayo, J.G., Boyd, M.R. (1987): Novel intrapulmonary model for orthotopic propagation of human lung cancers in athymic nude mice. Cancer Res. 47:5132–5140.

Pimm, M.V., Baldwin, R.W. (1987): Comparative biodistribution and rates of catabolism of radiolabelled anti-CEA monclonal antibody in control immunoglobulin in nude mice with human tumour xenografts showing specific antibody localization. Eur. J. Nucl. Med. 13:258–263.

Pimm, M.V., Perkins, A.C., Baldwin, R.W. (1985): Differences in tumour and normal tissue concentrations of iodine and indium labelled monoclonal antibody. II Biodistribution studies in mice with human tumour xenografts. Eur. J. Nucl. Med. 11:300–304.

Pimm, M.V., Pascoe, W., Robins, R.A., Price, M.R., Baldwin, R.W. (1986): Effect of protein mass on the pharmacokinetics and tumour discrimination of a murine monoclonal antibody in a rat mammary tumour model IRCS Med. Sci. 14:876–877.

Pressman, D., Korngold, L. (1953): The in vivo localization of anti-Wagner osteogenic sarcoma antibodies. Cancer 6:619–613.

Pressman, D., Day, E.D., Blau, M. (1957): The use of paired labeling in the determination of tumor-localizing antibodies. Cancer Res. 17:845–850.

Rosebrough, S.F., Grossman, Z.D., McAfee, J.G., Kudryk, B.J., Subramanian, G., Ritter-Hrncirik, C.A., Witanowski, L.S., Tillapaugh-Fay, G., Urrutia, E., Zapf-Longo, C. (1988): Thrombus imaging with indium-111 and iodine-131-labeled fibrin specific monoclonal antibody and its F(ab')$_2$ and Fab fragments. J. Nucl. Med. 29:1212–1222.

Rubin, R.H., Young, L.S., Hansen, P., Edelman, M., Wilkinson, R., Nelles, M.J., Callahen, R., Khaw, B.A., Strauss, H.W. (1988): Specific and non-specific imaging of localized Fisher Immunotype I Pseudomonas aeruginosa infection with radiolabeled monoclonal antibody. J. Nucl. Med. 29:651–656.

Sands, H., Jones, P.L. (1987): Methods for the study of the metabolism of radiolabeled monoclonal antibodies by liver and tumour. J. Nucl. Med. 28:390–398.

Shah, S.A., Gallagher, B.M., Sands, H. (1985): Radioimmunodetection of small human tumour xenografts in spleen of athymic mice by monoclonal antibody. Cancer Res. 45:5824–5829.

Shah, S.A., Gallagher, B.M., Sands, H. (1987): Lymphoscintigraphy of human carcinoma metastasis in athymic mice by use of radioiodinated B72.3 monoclonal antibody. J. Natl. Cancer Inst. 78:1069–1077.

Sands, H., Jones, P.L., Neacy, W.P., Shah, S.A., Gallagher, B.M. (1986): Site-related differences in the localization of the monoclonal antibody OX7 in SL2 and SL1 lymphomas. Cancer Immunol. Immunother. 22:169–175.

Shorthouse, A.J., Smyth, J.F., Steel, G.G., Ellison, M., Mills, J., Peckham, M.J. (1980): The human tumour xenograft—A valid model in experimental chemotherapy? Br. J. Surg. 67:715–722.

Som, P., Oster, Z.H., Zamora, P.O., Yamamoto, K., Sacker, D.F., Brill, A.B., Newall, K.D., Rhodes, B.A. (1986): Radioimaging of experimental thrombi in dogs using technetium-99m-labeled monoclonal antibody fragments reactive with human platelets. J. Nucl. Med. 27:1315–1320.

Steel, G.G., Courtney, V.D., Rostam, A. (1978). Improved immune-suppression techniques for the xenografting of human tumours. Br. J. Cancer 37:224–230.

Waldman, T.A., Strober, W. (1969): Metabolism of immunoglobulins. Prog. Allergy 13:1–110.

Ward, B.G., Wallace, K., Shepherd, J.H., Balkwill, F.R. (1987): Intraperitoneal xenografts of human epithelial ovarian cancer in nude mice. Cancer Res. 47:2662–2667.

Wochner, R.D., Adatepe, M., Van Amberg, A., Potchen, E.J. (1970): A new method for estimation of plasma volume with the use of the distribution space of indium-113m-transferrin. J. Lab. Clin. Med. 75:711–720.

4 Administration of Antibodies to Patients

INTRODUCTION

Although many of the early claims regarding the targeting capabilities of monoclonal antibodies have not been realised, these molecules presently represent a unique range of agents with a vast clinical potential. The full potential is still some way off, particularly regarding the use of antibodies for therapy, but despite an initially long gestation period we are now entering a phase of demonstrated clinical value. The use of *in vitro* assays for monitoring the level of serum antigen levels and of immunohistology for the classification of tissue sections is having a dramatic effect on departments of biochemistry and pathology. In comparison, the *in vivo* use of antibodies has been more restricted to specialised centres with the technical support necessary for purification, sterility testing, radiolabelling, and imaging. In addition, the *in vivo* administration of antibodies (which in the past have mainly been in the form of murine immunoglobulins) has been subject to rigorous ethical control and licensing by National Departments of Health. At the present time a number of biotechnology and radiopharmaceutical companies are producing antibodies for *in vivo* use, although most clinical studies have been restricted to research establishments as part of research programmes. The late 1980s and early 1990s have been a period of data collection, as antibodies with a definable clinical role are sifted out and assessed. The selection of antibodies suitable for clinical use is generally a slow process, with only a fraction (probably <5%) of the antibodies generated reaching a stage when they are ready for clinical use. This represents an enormous volume of *in vitro* work in the laboratory. Following production of a suitable antibody-producing clone, the antibody must be purified, tested for pyrogenicity and toxicity, and then radiolabelled, whilst preserving immunoreactivity as described in Chapters 1 and 2, this volume. Even after biodistribution studies and imaging studies, first in animals and subsequently in patients, the antibody may not be considered of any clinical value. Assuming the antibody is shown to be of clinical potential, a large amount of investment is necessary in order to provide the basic clinical data required for product registration by the licensing authorities. Only after all these stages have been completed is the antibody considered to be suitable for commercial sale as a clinical product.

For many years radiopharmaceuticals were partially exempt from many of the requirements applied to other standard pharmaceuticals in Western Europe. This was not the situation in the United States, however, where products have been strictly controlled by the Food and Drug Administration (FDA). The restrictions in the United States have had an adverse effect on the amount of clinical research undertaken, whereas in Europe the 1980s saw an increasing amount of clinical work which led to a number of antibodies proving to be of clinical value. The regulatory restrictions in the United States have resulted in a number of companies showing interest in carrying out clinical trials in Europe. By 1992 the situation will change to some degree and commercial production and sale of all radiopharmaceutical products in Europe will be regulated by the European Commission. The commercial production of radiopharmaceuticals based on monoclonal antibodies represents a particular challenge to radiopharmaceutical companies, since they are being forced to develop or adopt entirely new technologies for ensuring the purity, identity, and sterility of products. Most large pharmaceutical companies have some interests or subsidiaries with interests in monoclonal antibodies. In some cases the investment required has proved to be prohibitive. For example, Amersham International plc UK closed the development and production of the platelet specific murine antibody (P256), as it was envisaged that an investment of the order of £6 million would be required before a commercially viable

product would be available. Other companies such as Centocor are stepping up their commitment to the development of antibody based products by specialising in the new technologies, their aim being to produce a range of clinically useful products. Centocor Europe was the first company in Europe to secure a product licence for a monoclonal antibody based radiopharmaceutical. Myoscint (R11D10) is an antibody specific for myosin and may be used for the detection of myocardial infarct and the assessment of cardiac transplant rejection (see Chapter 7, this volume).

This chapter outlines some of the basic considerations for the clinical administration of antibodies and provides some of the information necessary for generating protocols for clinical studies.

CRITERIA FOR HUMAN ADMINISTRATION

Before an antibody may be considered suitable for human administration it must satisfy a number of criteria. The main criteria for the production and testing of antibodies were given in Chapter 1, this volume. Further guidance is provided in the "Operation Manual for Control of Production, Preclinical Toxicology and Phase 1 Trials of Anti-Tumour Antibodies and Drug Conjugates," which was published in the British Journal of Cancer (1986). In addition to testing for toxicity, pyrogenicity, and sterility, it is necessary to determine whether the material to be administered will have any potential effect (beneficial or adverse) on the patient or on the patient's immune system, with particular regard for the patients clinical condition. Pilot research studies and Phase 1 clinical trials are generally carried out on the assumption that administration of the material may result in some benefit to the patient, by virtue of additional diagnostic information or a possible therapeutic effect. However, since in most cases the aim of the trial is to examine the performance of the material, any possible effects will not be evident until after the material has been administered. In some cases this may be many months after the initial administration. For example, one of the main adverse effects of the administration of murine monoclonal antibody to patients has been the immune reaction and the formation of human anti-mouse antibody. In some cases this has led to problems with subsequent administration of antibody to the same patients some years later (see Chapter 6, this volume). As with the clinical introduction of any new drug, it is important that adverse reactions are recorded and reported to the appropriate authorities. For example, in Europe national schemes exist for reporting adverse effects of radiopharmaceuticals. In the United States similar arrangements exist with the Food and Drug Administration. In general terms, the administration of murine antibody to patients is considered safe, and from the many thousands of administrations throughout Europe alone, reported reactions are of the order of 1 in 1000, this being less than with many conventional pharmaceuticals.

LEGAL AND ETHICAL CONSIDERATIONS

Once an antibody or conjugate has been considered safe for clinical use, the ultimate decision rests with the physician taking clinical responsibility for the patient. The normal situation in research clinics is for the research proposals to be submitted to a hospital ethical committee. In this way, the responsibility for clinical trials is shared after due consideration of all perti-

nent information regarding the materials or drugs under evaluation, the methods of clinical evaluation, and the analysis of results.

It is often insisted that patients give informed consent prior to being entered into a trial, and many patients will agree on the basis that, even if the procedure does not have any beneficial effect on them personally, the information obtained may be of value to other patients at some time in the future. Individual circumstances vary between the various groups of antibodies currently of interest. Clearly different criteria will apply for, example, with regard to the investigation of malignant and non-malignant conditions. In general terms, as with any diagnostic investigation, any possible risks from the procedure must be balanced against the benefits of additional clinical information which may result from the study. Further discussion regarding the ethical considerations of the *in vivo* use of monoclonal antibodies is out of the scope of this book.

Additional regulations apply throughout the various countries of Europe and America. These normally take the form of clinical trial certificates or exemption certificates as appropriate. In the case of antibodies incorporated into radiopharmaceuticals, additional certificates are often a legal necessity. For example, in the UK, for the administration of a radioactive compound, a physician experienced in the use of radionuclides must hold a certificate from the Administration of Radioactive Substances Advisory Committee (ARSAC), which is issued through the Department of Health. Applications must state the radionuclide, amount of radioactivity to be administered, the nature of the compound, and an effective radiation dose equivalent following administration of the material. The application must also give details of the patient group to be studied and any control subjects. It must also be approved by the local head of scientific services and the Radiation Protection Advisor. Once granted, the certificate is then valid for a two-year period of research, or for a defined number of subjects, and permits the work to be carried out on the premises specified. Similar arrangements exist in most other Western countries.

Specific Regulations Within the United States

In July 1983 the office of Biologics Research and Review Centre for Drugs and Biologics of the American FDA drafted the "Points to Consider in the Manufacture of Monoclonal Antibodies for Human Use." This document was subsequently revised and updated in 1987 (Centre for Drugs and Biologics, FDA 1987). The document covers the development of murine monoclonal antibodies in the United States and gives details of the Office of Biologic's expectations regarding filing of Notices of Claimed Investigational Exemption (INDs) and product licensing. A further document "Points to Consider in the Characterisation of Cell Lines Used to Produce Biologicals" was issued from the FDA in 1987. This document emphasises the identification and characterisation cell substrate and testing of the bulk and final product. A summary of the basic requirements for submission to the FDA is given in Table 4.1.

Specific Regulations Within Europe

In Europe, the Commission of the European Communities set up an ad hoc working party on biotechnology/pharmacology which drafted notes for guidance on "Radiopharmaceuticals Based on Monoclonal Antibodies," which were first published in 1988. The initial draft of this document introduced strict controls on the characterisation and production of monoclonal antibodies for commercial use. Such was the impact of this document that the authorities in certain member countries immediately prohibited clinical trials with antibodies produced by commercial laboratories. For example, clinical research using Sorin melanoma antibody was prohibited in hospitals within the Netherlands. Universities and research institutes which had allowed the use of monoclonal antibodies in local trials felt the need to protect themselves with insurance cover for such trials. The insurance companies subsequently required stricter control than had hitherto been required. This added significantly to the difficulty and cost of producing materials suitable for clinical trials.

The third draft of the European guidelines was released in October 1989 via the Office for Official Publications in the European Communities (Luxembourg). This now specifically states that "the guidelines are intended to be used by manufacturers submitting applications for market authorization. They are not intended as guidelines for non-commercial producers." At the present time these guidelines are advisory and not mandatory. The guidelines are similar in form to those of the US Food and Drug administration, although not as stringent. They stress the importance of good manufacturing practice and comprehensive documentation regarding source material, production facilities, radionuclide labelling procedures and dosimetry, specifications and quality control, pre-clinical safety testing, toxicity testing, pharmacodynamics, and pharmacokinetics. Of interest is a list of information which must be included on the pack-

TABLE 4.1. A Summary of Information Required by the US Food and Drug
Administration Prior to Submission for IND

1. Characterisation of hybridoma cell lines	4. Tests on unprocessed and final bulk lots
Origin of cell lines	Bacteria, fungi, mycoplasma and viruses
Species, animal strain and tissue of origin	Immunological specificity
Identification of immunogen	Detection of aggregation, denaturation
Immunisation scheme	and specificity
Screening procedure	Degree of homogeneity of fragment
Cell cloning procedures	preparations
	Immunoglobulin class and subclass
2. Production procedure	Isoelectric focusing pattern
Tissue culture procedure	Sterility
Supplier, genotype and husbandry of	Polynucleotide contamination
animals used	Potency
Production, harvesting and handling of	Electrophoretic migration
ascites	Protein contamination
Steps taken to control viral, bacterial,	Pyrogenicity
fungal and mycoplasmal contamination	Stability
3. Purification procedures	5. Preclinical toxicity tests
Size exclusion chromatography	Pharmacological safety
Affinity chromatography	(immunoconjugates and immunotoxins)
Ion-exchange chromatography	*In vitro* cross reactivity
Ultracentrifugation	
Physical and chemical treatments such as	
pH or temperature variation, exposure	
to chelators or solvents	

age insert of antibodies intended for clinical use. This is reproduced in Table 4.2 for the benefit of future users of commercial antibody products in Europe.

BIODISTRIBUTION OF MONOCLONAL ANTIBODIES IN PATIENTS

Published clinical trials with monoclonal antibodies have reported widely varying amounts of protein administered for imaging studies. These have generally varied from less than 100 μg to in excess of 50 mg. In some cases additional doses of non-labelled antibody (30 to 50 mg) have been given concurrently with the radiolabelled dose, mainly with the aim of increasing the target to non-target uptake ratio. The administration of cold antibody prior to the administration of radiolabelled antibody has been advocated on the hypothesis that the cold antibody will saturate the antigen sites in normal tissues, which will be fewer in number than those in target tissues. In theory, this then gives a greater opportunity for the radiolabelled antibody to localise in the abnormal tissues where the number of antigen sites are higher. The main disadvantage of this approach is that the administration of higher amounts of antibody is more likely to result in increased

TABLE 4.2. Information Required to be Supplied With Commercial Antibody Products
by the Commission of the European Community

1. The name of the product and a description of its use.

2. A list of the contents of the kit.

3. The name and the address of the manufacturer of the kit.

4. Identification and specifications concerning the radiolabelling materials that can be used to prepare the radiopharmaceutical.

5. Directions for preparing the radiopharmaceutical including range of activity and volume and a statement of the storage requirements for the prepared pharmaceutical.

6. A statement of the useful life of the prepared pharmaceutical.

7. Indications and contraindications in respect of the prepared pharmaceutical.

8. Precautions to be taken by the user and the patient during the preparation and use of the product, and special precautions for the disposal of the container and any unused contents.

9. Where applicable, and pharmacology and toxicology of the prepared radiopharmaceutical including the route of elimination and effective half-life.

10. The radiation dose of the patient from the prepared radiopharmaceutical.

11. A statement of recommended use for the prepared radiopharmaceutical and the recommended dose.

12. A statement of the route of administration of the prepared radiopharmaceutical, and

13. If necessary, a recommendation that the radiochemical purity of the prepared radiopharmaceutical must be checked prior to administration. In such cases methods and specifications must be given.

sensitisation of the patient, thus reducing the clinical use of the technique for diagnosis.

When radiolabelled murine monoclonal antibody is injected intravenously into patients for immunoscintigraphy, its blood survival and biodistribution might be expected to be similar to that in mice. That is, one might expect a rapid extravasation phase, during which the antibody passes partly into extravascular tissue fluid, and then a slower phase representing the actual catabolism of the antibody, during which time the proportion of remaining antibody, intra- and extravascular, remains constant. It is during this distribution and catabolism that specific antigen recognition in the target lesion takes place, and there is a build up of target to non-target distribution of the tracer. When the optimum balance between target to non-target ratio, blood clearance, and overall catabolism of the monoclonal antibody (and clearance of breakdown products) has been attained, imaging of the lesion might be expected to be achieved at its best.

While some monoclonal antibodies do show the expected pattern of biodistribution, others do not, even though they may still be effective in imaging. It is only now becoming realised that there are a number of factors which can perturb the biodistribution of a monoclonal antibody away

TABLE 4.3. Factors Influencing the Biodistribution of Monoclonal Antibodies

1. Circulating antigen may be present released from the target lesion. This antigen may form complexes with the monoclonal antibody, encouraging its liver clearance and/or circulating antibody may not be able to recognise target tissue.

2. The target antigen may be expressed in some normal tissue. Images may show some uptake of tracer into normal organ(s), but this might be dose-related so that true target discrimination improves with antibody dose.

3. Antibody may interact, specifically or non-specifically with blood elements. This could result in rapid clearance of the antibody, compromising target recognition, and with possible deleterious effects on the patient.

4. Antibodies present in the patient's plasma may complex with the monoclonal antibody. This could prevent effective target localisation of the antibody, and clearance of the complexes could produce image artefacts.

from that expected from the simple model (Table 4.3). Clearly, therefore, some study of the blood kinetics, catabolism, etc., of a monoclonal antibody during the early stages of its evaluation in patients can provide data which is valuable in understanding the imaging characteristics of that particular antibody. Moreover, as we will see below, such data can sometimes provide new insights into the nature and expression of the target antigen defined by the monoclonal antibody and hitherto not appreciated from pre-clinical in vitro or experimental animal studies. Such determinations should form an important part of the evaluation of new antibodies.

BLOOD CLEARANCE KINETICS

Table 4.4 summarises some of the reported blood clearance half times of monoclonal antibodies and their fragments. This shows, where available, the first and second phase half times, although often fulltime course data is not available. It should be borne in mind that the representation of the clearance form the blood of monoclonal antibodies as having two distinct phases is a somewhat idealised view. Often

the clearance is more complex and, if expressed really accurately, might have several phases. Nevertheless, an overview of the available data in this way is probably useful, since it gives some idea of the usual range of antibody clearance kinetics to allow some comparison with other antibodies.

Where data is available, the first phase half time with intact antibody is within the range of 11–15 hours, followed by a second phase of between 18 and 44 hours. With $F(ab)_2$, a first phase of less than 2 hours has been reported, followed by a second with about 20 hour half time, and similar values were obtained with Fab fragment in the one reported study. Figure 4.1 shows some of the authors' studies with the 791T/36 monoclonal antibody. I-131 labelled intact antibody had a mean initial half time of 0.62 days, followed by a second phase of 1.85 day half time. Similar results were seen with the same antibody labelled with In-111. In contrast, with the Fab fragment, the initial half time was only 0.2 days, and the second phase 0.78 days.

Manipulation of the data of the second and first phases of these types of blood clearance curves enable some calculation

TABLE 4.4. Some Examples of Blood Clearance Half-Times of Radiolabelled Monoclonal Antibodies in Patients Injected for Immunoscintigraphy[a]

Antibody	Disease	Radiolabel	Mean half-times (hours)		Intra-vascular fraction	Authors
			First phase	Second phase		
791T/36	Colorectal, ovarian carcinoma, osteosarcoma	I-131	14.9	44.4	0.43	Pimm et al. (1985)
		In-111	11.0	33.6	0.43	
791T/36-Fab	Colorectal, ovarian carcinoma, osteosarcoma	I-131	4.8	18.7	0.18	Pimm et al. (1985)
HMFG2	Ovarian carcinoma	I-131	NR[b]	38	NR	Ward et al. (1987)
HMFG2	Ovarian, breast, gastrointestinal tumours	I-123	NR	18	NR	Epenetos et al. (1982)
B72.3	Colon carcinoma	I-131	NR	60–70[c]	NR	Carrasquillo et al. (1988)
19.9-F(ab)$_2$	Colorectal, ovarian, lung, pancreatic carcinoma	In-111	2	19	0.38	Hnatowich et al. (1985)
OC-125-F(ab)$_2$	Ovarian carcinoma	In-111	NR	21	1.0	Hnatowich et al. (1987)
96.5	Melanoma	In-111	NR	32	NR	Rosenblum et al. (1985)
ZME018	Melanoma	In-111	NR	24	NR	Lamki et al. (1987)
ZCE025	Colon carcinoma	In-111	NR	27	NR	Lamki et al. (1987)
PAY-276	Prostate carcinoma	In-111	NR	22	NR	Lamki et al. (1987)
ID4	Thyroid tumour	I-123	NR	24	NR	Shepherd et al. (1985)

[a] All antibodies were injected intravenously.
[b] NR Not reported.
[c] Calculated from data in the cited paper.

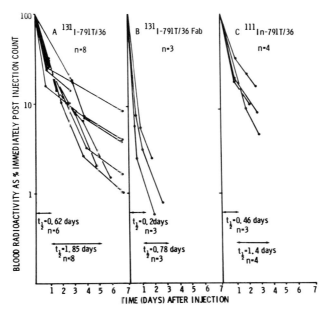

Fig. 4.1. Blood survival of the monoclonal antibody 791T/36 after intravenous injection into patients with colorectal cancer. A blood sample was taken within minutes of injection and daily for up to seven days. Note the similar clearance curves for both In-111- and I-131-labelled antibody, but the quite different profile for Fab. (Reproduced from Pimm et al., J. Nuc . Med. 26:1011–1023, 1985, with permission of the Society of Nuclear Medicine.)

of the proportion of the radiolabelled antibody, which is intravascular compared with that which is extravascular. An intravascular fraction of 0.43 for both I-131 and In-111 labelled intact 791T/36 antibody, and 0.18 for its Fab fragment, was obtained by the authors, while Hnatowich et al. (1985) reported 0.38 for $F(ab)_2$ fragment of 19.9 antibody.

It is a pity that more and fuller data is not available on the blood clearance kinetics of radiolabelled antibodies during immunoscintigraphy investigations since this would be especially valuable for estimating radiation absorbed doses. Simple blood sampling immediately after injection, at intervals of two or three hours over the first twelve hours, and then at daily interval for a few days, would provide valuable data on the biodistribution of antibod-

ies and how they are being catabolized. Simple assay of the radiolabel in a standard volume of blood (1 ml usually has an adequate count rate for counting in a conventional gamma counter) will allow construction of time activity curves for blood survival of the radiolabel. These figures can be related to the initial dose by reference to a sample of the injected material. The total blood volume of the patient can be calculated from weight and age by reference to standard physiological tables, and the proportion of the dose remaining in the whole circulation can also be determined.

EXCRETION OF RADIOLABELS

From some imaging studies the whole body retention of radiolabel has been calculated. This can be done from images themselves, especially when rectilinear scanners are used, and/or from the levels of radiolabel excreted in the urine. It might be expected from experimental animal studies (see Chapter 3, this volume) that radioiodines would be excreted following catabolism, and then the excretion half times would be similar to those of the catabolic phase blood clearance of the radioiodine. With radiometals, which are not readily excreted following antibody catabolism, excretion might be slower and not parallel to that of the blood clearance. The limited amount of available data (Table 4.5) indicate that this is in fact so. Thus with In-111-labelled antibodies, given either intraperitoneally or intravenously, excretion is slow, only a few percent of the dose being lost over several days. In some cases there may be a fairly rapid loss over the first few hours, but this is probably due to excretion of free DTPA-In-111 in the preparation, and subsequently loss is very slow. With I-131 labelled-antibodies, whole body survival half times are within the 40–80 hour range.

It is interesting to note here the long whole body retention times of radioindium from labelled antibodies compared with radioiodine, although the blood kinetics of the two sorts of labelled antibodies are very similar (Table 4.4). This sort of data substantiates what is seen in experimental models (Chapter 3, this volume) and should be borne in mind when considering the different imaging characteristics of radiometal compared with radioiodine labelled antibodies.

The radiolabel excreted in the urine is not predominantly associated with antibody or antibody fragments, as shown by its lack of precipitability with TCA or anti-Ig antiserum. With radioiodine labelled antibodies, the excreted radioiodine is as free iodide or iodotyrosine, while with radioindium labelled preparations the excreted material may be DTPA-In-111 or other low-molecular-weight materials.

THE CHARACTERISTICS OF CIRCULATING RADIOLABELLED MONOCLONAL ANTIBODY

If antibody injected intravenously is to localise in target lesions, it must survive in the circulation in an intact, immunologically active form. There are a few reports of some monoclonal antibodies reacting with blood cell elements sufficiently to perturb the imaging of target lesions. For example, Dillman et al. (1984), when using an anti-CEA antibody which was not CEA-specific and cross reacted with NCA expressed on circulating granulocytes, reported that there was such a binding of the antibody to the granulocytes as to prevent imaging of metastatic tumour. Such instances are fortunately rare, and indeed *in vitro* assessment of antibodies before clinical use should be able to identify such cross reactivities.

The Nature of Circulating Radiolabel

In other situations where the nature of blood-borne radiolabel has been assessed, the majority of the radiolabel is found in plasma and not associated with cellular elements. Relatively simple techniques are available to fractionate fresh blood into plasma, red cells, and leucocytes, the latter being separable into monocytes and granulocytes. For example, Figure 4.2 is an example of the authors' study (Powell et al., 1987) of the blood-borne I-131-labelled 791T/36 monoclonal antibody in patients undergoing immunoscintigraphy. Ninety percent or more of the radiolabel in blood

TABLE 4.5. Whole Body Retention of Radiolabels by Patients Undergoing Immunoscintigraphy

Antibody	Disease	Radiolabel	Route	Excretion	Measurement method	Authors
791T/36	Ovarian carcinoma	I-131	I.P.	Half time 42 hours	Urine counts	Perkins et al. (1989)
791T/36	Ovarian carcinoma	In-111	I.P.	4% in 4 days	Urine counts	
B72.3	Colon carcinoma	I-131	I.V.	Half time 82 hours	Probe counts and whole body scans	Carrasquillo et al. (1988)
19.9-F(ab)$_2$	Colorectal, ovarian, lung, pancreatic carcinoma	In-111	I.V.	Half time 160 hours	Whole body scans	Hnatowich et al. (1985)
96.5	Melanoma	In-111	I.V.	9% within 8 hours, then 5% within 40 hours	Urine counts	Rosenblum et al. (1985)
HMFG2	Ovarian carcinoma	I-123	I.P.	Half time 50 hours	Urine counts	Ward et al. (1987)

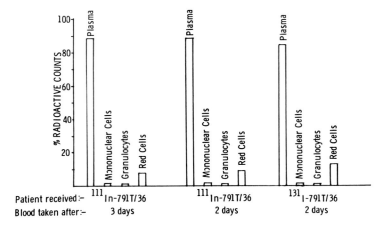

Fig. 4.2. Distribution of radioactivity in elements of the blood in patients with ovarian carcinoma who had been injected with labelled 791T/36 monoclonal antibody. Note that the majority of the radiolabel is in plasma immediately after injection and this is maintained for at least two days, with very little association with white cells, although about 10% is recovered in the red cell fraction. (Reproduced from Powell et al., Am. J. Obstet. Gynecol. 157:28–34, 1987, with permission of the publisher.)

samples taken several days after intravenous injection was in plasma. Where data is available it suggests that other antibodies too survive in the circulation in the plasma rather than associated with blood cells. For example, with In-111-labelled OC125 antibody, Hnatowich et al. (1987) found that less than 3% of the radioactivity associated with blood cells for at least 96 hours after injection.

The tests used to determine the quality and immunological reactivity of radiolabelled monoclonal antibody preparations before their injection (see Chapter 2, this volume) can also be used to test the nature and immunological function of the plasma-borne radiolabelled material surviving in the circulation. For example, precipitation test with agents such as TCA or anti-mouse Ig antiserum usually shows that the majority of circulating material is still attached not only to protein but to the mouse monoclonal antibody itself.

Analysis of the molecular size of circulating material can be carried out by gel filtration chromatography or HPLC. With radioiodine labelled antibody this often shows that the molecular size of the circulating material is unchanged, i.e., the circulating monoclonal antibody is still in its original form. Figure 4.3 shows an example from the authors' study with I-131-labelled 791T/36 monoclonal antibody. The elution profile from Sephacryl S-300 of the labelled antibody was virtually identical when added to normal human plasma, or when plasma was from a patient injected two days before with the labelled preparation.

With Indium-111 labelled antibodies, radiolabel in the circulation is sometimes found in association with a lower molecular fraction of the plasma, and this is usually due to binding of the radiometal to plasma transferrin. Figure 4.4 shows another example from the authors' work with the 791T/36 monoclonal antibody. Here Sephacryl S-300 gel filtration of the In-111 labelled antibody added to normal plasma showed only one peak of eluted radiolabel. When plasma was taken from a patient three days after intravenous injection of

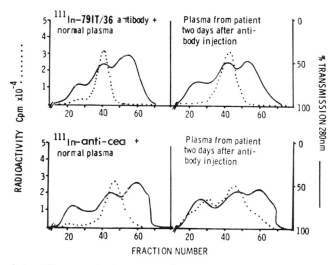

Fig. 4.3. Examples of the differences in the nature of circulating radiolabelled antibody depending on the presence of circulating antigen. Two patients with colorectal cancer were injected intravenously with In-111-labelled 791T/36 or In-111-labelled anti-CEA monoclonal antibodies. Prior addition of samples of each labelled antibody to normal plasma and chromatography on Sephacryl S-300 showed both preparations were homogeneous, radiolabel eluting with the second plasma protein peak in the expected 150,000 dalton region. When plasma taken from the patients two days after injection was similarly examined by gel filtration, that from the patient given 791T/36 showed circulating radiolabel virtually indistinguishable from the initial preparation. In contrast that from the patient given anti-CEA monoclonal antibody showed about 50% of the radioindium now eluting at a higher molecular weight, due to the formation in the circulation of immune complexes with CEA present before the injection. (From the authors' studies).

antibody, there was a "shoulder" in the elution profile, some of the In-111 eluting from the column at a lower molecular weight (the molecular weight of transferrin is 88,000 daltons). Whether this sort of process represents only transchelation from the antibody to the transferrin actually in the circulation or whether transferrin can also pick up radioindium from sites of the antibody catabolism is not known. The plasma half time of radioindium labelled transferrin has been reported to be only six hours (Wochner et al., 1970), shorter than that of most antibodies or even their fragments, and therefore it is unlikely that labelled transferrin will become the dominant labelled protein in the plasma; generally this transchelation has not been a problem in imaging with In-111-labelled antibodies.

Immunological Reactivity of Circulating Antibody

If radiolabelled antibody is to recognise target lesions, not only must it survive in the circulation long enough, but it must also retain its immunological activity. The antigen binding potential of the plasma-borne radiolabel can be assessed in antigen binding assays in the same way as the initial labelled preparation using appropriate forms of the antigen such a tumour cell suspensions in the case of anti-tumour antibodies. There are only a few reported studies in this field, but where it has been assessed, the circulating radiolabelled antibody can still bind to target antigen. For example, Hnatowich et al. (1985, 1987), with both In-111-labelled 19-9 antibody in patients with colorectal carcinoma and OC-125 antibody in those with ovarian car-

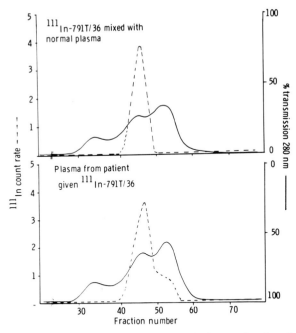

Fig. 4.4. Detection of *in vivo* transchelation of In-111 from labelled monoclonal antibody to serum transferrin. The top panel shows the elution profile from Sephacryl S-300 of In-111-labelled 791T/36 monoclonal antibody added to normal human plasma, the radiolabel eluting as a distinct peak. Plasma taken from a patient with ovarian cancer who had been injected 3 days earlier with the labelled antibody was similarly run on Sephacryl S-300 (bottom panel). Although the position of the major peak of radioindium is unchanged there is some tracer in a lower molecular weight form, as a result of its attachment to transferrin. (Reproduced from Powell et al., Am. J. Obstet. Gynecol. 157:28–34, 1987, with permission of the publisher.)

cinoma, have shown that up to at least 96 hours after injection the circulating radiolabel can bind to immunoabsorbants of the appropriate antigens. In some patients injected with these antibodies there was a slow decline in the proportion of the radiolabel capable of binding to antigen. This was seen even more so in studies by the authors, with the 791T/36 monoclonal antibody labelled with either I-131 and In-111 in patients with colorectal carcinoma where one or two days after injection the proportion of radioactivity detected which was capable of binding to tumour target cells was only about half of that in the injected preparations. Nevertheless this was specific antigen recognition, and the circu-

lating radiolabel did not bind to other tumour cells which did not produce the target antigen. The reason for this type of decline in immunological activity is unclear. It could be due to some denaturation of the antibody during its circulation.

The Influence of Circulating Antigen

One important factor which could reduce the antigen binding activity of circulating radiolabelled monoclonal antibody is its neutralisation by antigen which has been shed into the blood-stream from the target lesion. The presence of circulating antigen detectable with monoclonal antibodies has been examined particularly in cancer patients because such serum markers, detectable in *in vitro* assays, may be useful in their own right in tumour diagnosis or prognosis. In the case of some monoclonal antibodies which have been used for immunoscintigraphy, circulating antigen is not found. For example, with the 96.5 anti-melanoma antibody, the antigen with which it reacts was not detectable in the serum of the majority of patients with melanoma undergoing immunoscintigraphy (Murray et al., 1985). Similarly the antigen identified by the 791T/36 monoclonal antibody, which has been used for imaging colorectal and ovarian carcinomas, is not detectable in the plasma of these patients (Pimm et al., 1985), and this cannot explain the reduced immunological reactivity of circulating antibody in patients undergoing immunoscintigraphy.

However, some other monoclonal antibody-defined antigens are present in patients' plasma and can form immune complexes with radiolabelled antibody. This was seen very early on in the development of immunoscintigraphy with anti-CEA antibodies when it was shown by techniques such as gel filtration chromatography that the circulating radiolabel was in a high-molecular-weight complex. Figure 4.3 is an example comparing In-111 labelled 791T/36 monoclonal antibody with In-111-labelled anti-CEA monoclonal antibody in patients with colorectal carcinoma. With 791T/36 the elution profile of the radiolabel does not change after two days in the patient's circulation, while with the anti-CEA, part of the radiolabel now runs in a higher molecular weight, as complexes with CEA.

It was shown in the early studies by Mach et al. (1981) that the proportion of the anti-CEA antibody dose going into such complexes increased with the level of

CEA originally in the circulation. With the OC-125 antibody in ovarian cancer patients, analysis of plasma samples shows the gradual appearance of radiolabel in high molecular form, although with this antibody the proportion of circulating radiolabel present in high molecular weight form did not correlate well with the initial plasma antigen levels (Hnatowich et al., 1987).

Surprisingly, these sort of complexes between monoclonal antibodies and antigen are not cleared into the liver or spleen as might be expected, but seem to be retained in the circulation. What is even more surprising about this formation of circulating complexes is that it does not seem generally to interfere with successful immunodetection of tumours, and certainly the efficiency of tumour imaging with OC-125 and anti-CEA antibodies seems to be unrelated to the circulating antigen level or degree of complex formation. A similar conclusion has been drawn about the B72.3 monoclonal antibody in imaging colorectal carcinoma, where the TAG-72 antigen is present at elevated levels in about 60% of patients, but this does not interfere with tumour imaging (Colcher et al., 1987).

It has been suggested that the efficient detection of tumours in spite of the vast majority of radiolabelled antibody present in the circulation as complexes with antigen could be due to the monoclonal antibodies having a higher affinity for tissue-bound antigen than for the soluble plasma-borne antigen. It is possible that the antibody can dissociate from the antigen in the circulation and react with that in the tumour. With anti-CEA antibodies, Bosslet et al. (1988) have definitely shown higher affinity of binding to cell-associated CEA than to CEA present in patients' plasma, and have suggested that this is due to conformational changes in the circulating CEA.

This is obviously an area in which further investigation is required, because it cannot be assumed that all antibodies will show this phenomenon. For example, Bosslet et al. also showed that other antibodies which reacted with CEA, but which were not CEA-specific and also reacted with NCA, did not show this effect and reacted equally well with both plasma-borne and cell surface CEA. It is feasible that some tumour-specific monoclonal antibodies might be prevented from target localisation by complex formation in the circulation, and in some cases these complexes might not survive in the circulation but might be cleared, probably to liver or spleen. Information on the levels of circulating antigen and some examination of the nature of the circulating radiolabelled antibody shortly after injection would be advisable in the early stages of clinical evaluation of any new antibody.

The Influence of Antibody Dose

In the early days of immunoscintigraphy low doses of radiolabelled monoclonal antibody were used, often less than one milligram. As long as sufficient radiolabel can be attached to this amount of antibody, the advantages of using low doses are obvious; the antibody preparations go further, and any possible side effects in the patients and/or generation of antibody responses to the monoclonal antibody are minimised.

Subsequently it was definitely shown with some antibodies that increasing the dose of antibody, with a constant amount of radiolabel, has no beneficial effect on imaging efficiency. For example, with the B72.3 antibody against colorectal carcinoma, a range of doses of between 0.16 mg and 20 mg all had the same blood clearance kinetics and tumour image detection rates (Colcher et al., 1987; Carrasquillo et al., 1988). This is one of the antibodies where patients had circulating antigen, and the finding of no relationship between antibody dose and blood kinetics and image quality added further weight to the argument that circulating antigen need not necessarily adversely affect immunoscintigraphy.

However, with some monoclonal antibodies it has been known for some time that imaging efficiency is dose-related, but the reasons for this are only now becoming clear. With the 96.5 monoclonal antibody in melanoma, Murray et al. (1985) reported imaging only two of twenty-three (9%) metastatic sites with 1 mg of antibody with 75 MBq of In-111, but nine out of twelve (75%) with 10 mg of antibody with the same amount of radioindium. Further studies by the same group of investigators has shown dose-related differences in the pharmacokinetics and image biodistribution with this antibody. In patients in whom administration of 1 mg of In-111 labelled antibody had been preceded by up to 39 mg of either unlabelled irrelevant monoclonal antibody or by unlabelled 96.5 monoclonal antibody, they showed that pretreatment with specific antibody reduced liver uptake of the radiolabel, but there was no effect with irrelevant immunoglobulin (Fig. 4.5). There was a significant drop in liver to heart ratios of radioactivity in the images of patients pre-treated with unlabelled antibody compared with those given the irrelevant immunoglobulin. Significant decreases in spleen to heart and bone to heart ratios were also observed.

The 96.5 monoclonal antibody is one for which circulating tumour antigen is not found in patients with melanoma, and the results of the dose response studies cannot be due to plasma-borne antigen perturbing

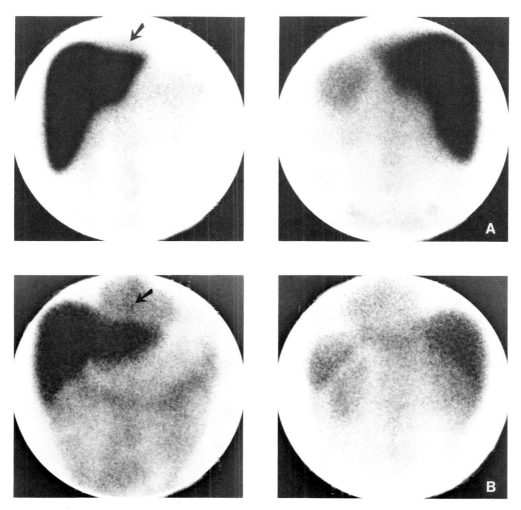

Fig. 4.5. A demonstration of the effect of the dose of monoclonal antibody on biodistribution seen by gamma scintigraphy. **A**: anterior **(left)** and posterior **(right)** 72 hour images of the abdomen of a patient receiving 19 mg of unlabelled irrelevant IgG2a monoclonal antibody one hour prior to the injection of 1 mg of the P96.5 IgG2a anti-melanoma monoclonal antibody labelled with In-111. There is a large amount of radioactivity in the liver compared to the heart (arrowed). **B**: similar views of a patient who received 19 mg of the unlabelled P96.5 anti-melanoma monoclonal antibody one hour before 1 mg of the same antibody labelled with In-111. Note that there is now significantly less radioactivity in the liver and greater in the heart compared to A. The interpretation here is that pre-treatment with P96.5 monoclonal antibody, but not non-specific antibody, saturated antigenic site in the liver capable of reacting with the P96.5 antibody, so that when In-111 labelled P96.5 was given uptake into the liver was reduced. (Reproduced from Murray et al., Cancer Res. 48:4417–4422, 1988, with permission of Dr J.L. Murray and The American Association for Cancer Research.)

biodistribution of low doses of monoclonal antibody. The most likely explanation of these findings is that the antigen identified by the monoclonal antibody is expressed in some normal tissues, particularly liver, spleen, and bone. As the antibody dose is increased, these sites become saturated while tumour uptake continues to increase, and consequently tumour discrimination improves. This phenomenon would perhaps be expected to be most obvious with the antibody In-111 labelled, because once localised in the liver, the radioindium released after catabolism would tend to be retained in this organ.

This effect is due to specific antigen recognition, and not due simply to saturation of sites with some natural propensity to take up mouse immunoglobulins because it could not produced when another but irrelevant monoclonal antibody, of the same isotype as the specific monoclonal antibody, was injected before the In-111-labelled specific antibody. This is an example of where the clinical imaging study can provide information on the target specificity of a monoclonal antibody hitherto unknown from *in vitro* examination of the antibody reactivity or its assessment in animal models.

A similar phenomenon has now been reported with at least three other monoclonal antibodies. Thus Lamki et al. (1988) carried out similar clinical studies with another antibody (ZME-018) against a different melanoma associated antigen, an anti-CEA antibody (ZCE-015) in colon carcinoma, and an anti-prostatic acid phosphatase antibody (PAY-276) in prostate cancer. In all cases, increasing the dose of In-111 labelled antibody reduced localisation in liver or spleen, increased blood pool activity, and increased tumour detection rates (Table 4.6).

As more and more antibodies are evaluated for immunoscintigraphy, the possibility of their showing this phenomenon should be borne in mind. It is possible that it will be more widely reported in the future. However, with antibodies which are already known to show this effect, the dose at which tumour imaging becomes maximal seems to vary from antibody to antibody (Table 4.6), and with other antibodies the optimum dose will probably have to be determined empirically. At the present time it is not clear whether there is an optimum dose of antibody for clinical imaging. Thomas et al. (1989) produced a compartmental model based on the affinity, molecular size, and injected dose. Their calculations suggest that the amount of antibody necessary for optimum targeting is more in the region of 100 mg than 100 μg and that it is necessary to calculate the optimum dose for each patient, based on the tumour burden (which should ideally be known beforehand), the antibody affinity, and the antigen levels in the patient.

Whether monoclonal antibodies which require doses as high as 40 or 50 mg to achieve effective imaging are acceptable for clinical use requires careful consideration. If low doses of these antibodies are used, a high proportion of the dose of radiolabel may be absorbed by normal tissues, and the dosimetry in these organs may be different from that expected, and, of course, imaging will not be very efficient. If high doses are given, this is expensive in terms of antibody, and any side effects due to adverse reactions and the development by the patient of antibodies to the monoclonal antibody could be increased.

RADIATION DOSIMETRY

The aim of any radionuclide investigation is to achieve the desired clinical result with the minimum radiation exposure to the patient. The patient's exposure will de-

TABLE 4.6. The Effect of Monoclonal Antibody Doses
on Detection Rates for Tumour Metastases

Antibody	Disease	Detection rates (%) of doses of			
		5 mg	10 mg	20 mg	40 mg
PAY-276	Prostate cancer	10	13	29	53
ZCE-025	Colon cancer	16	29	35	77
ZME-018	Melanoma	29	65	65	68

Data taken from Lamki et al. (1988).
Twenty patients were studied with each In-11-labelled antibody, there being five at each dose level. There were between 10 and 100 known metastatic sites in each group.

pend upon the radionuclide employed as the label, the amount of administered radioactivity, and the nature of the antibody preparation used, i.e., immunoglobulin class or subclass, fragmentation, and antigen and cross-reacting antigen recognition. These factors are crucial since the form of the antibody preparation, its binding properties, and the method of conjugation will affect the *in vivo* biodistribution, pharmacokinetics, and excretion pattern of the radiolabel. The physical factors affecting the internal radiation dosimetry of radiolabelled antibodies have been mentioned previously in Chapter 2, this volume. Values for the equilibrium-absorbed dose constants for the main radionuclides used in immunoscintigraphy are given in Table 4.7. To minimise the absorbed dose for diagnostic studies it is desirable to chose a radionuclide with pure gamma emission and a short physical half-life. Similarly the selection of an antibody with a short biological half-life will also minimise the absorbed radiation dose. For intact mouse IgG the biological half-life is about 2–3 days, whilst for Fab and F(ab')$_2$ fragments it is the order of about ½ day (see earlier sections in this chapter). However, the radiation dosimetry depends upon the

metabolic pathway of the conjugate and the subsequent physiological fate of the radionuclide (Pimm et al., 1985, Perkins and Pimm, 1985).

The magnitude of the radiation dose is generally based on the absorbed fraction method of calculation. This approach is internationally recognised and has been adopted by the Medical Internal Radiation Dose Committee (MIRD) of the Society of Nuclear Medicine and the International Commission on Radiological Protection (ICRP). Prior to initial studies in man it is often necessary to obtain information on radiation dosimetry from animal studies, although the direct extrapolation of animal data may not be accurate when applied to man. More accurate dosimetry calculations may be made following initial administrations to patients. It follows that the protocols for initial clinical trials should be designed so that measurements are taken, in order that more accurate information on the biodistribution and radiation dosimetry may be obtained. This information should then be made available to the National Licensing Authorities and will in turn aid in the design of future trials. The dosimetry calculation should be based on all target organ and whole body biodistri-

TABLE 4.7. Physical Characteristics and Absorbed Dose Constants
for Radionuclides Suitable for Antibody Imaging

Radionuclide	T1/2 physical	Decay mode	Whole body equilibrium absorbed dose constant kgGy/MBqh
123-1	13 h	Electron capture	0.14
131-I	8.0 d	β-emission	0.45
111-In	67 h	Electron capture	0.33
67 Ga	78 h	Electron capture	0.11
99mTc	6.0 h	Isometric transition	0.14

butions, with additional radiation estimation to radiosensitive tissues such as the haematopoietic system, gonads, and the lens of the eye. It is also important to consider any possible change in radiation dosimetry due to any alteration in the biodistribution which may occur in certain pathological conditions. Examples of radiation doses resulting from the administration of selected radiolabelled antibody preparations are given in Table 4.8. Further information on the relative absorbed radiation doses of different radiolabelled antibody preparations has been published by Britton et al., 1989.

IMAGING PROTOCOLS

With the range of In-111-, I-123-, and Tc-99m-labelled antibodies that are currently available, imaging procedures are reasonably straightforward. Following administration of the radiolabelled antibody it is advisable to obtain a blood pool view within the first 30 minutes. In addition to confirming that the dose has been injected correctly, the blood pool images provide information on the vascular anatomy, and any gross abnormality, such as highly perfused regions or cystic areas,

may be identified. The timing of subsequent views will depend upon the antibody preparation, the radiolabel, and the pathology being investigated. Table 4.9 provides the basic information for devising protocols for clinical studies. It is not possible to be too prescriptive regarding the dose of antibody and the timing of imaging since these will depend upon the antibody being used and the pathology being studied.

PILOT STUDIES AND UNTOWARD FINDINGS

In order for an antibody to be selected for administration to patients, the vast amount of work associated with the preclinical selection and testing of that antibody will have indicated that the antibody offers clinical potential. Nevertheless, the true clinical value of an antibody will not be realised until it has been tested in patients. The first clinical use of a new antibody is a time of apprehension for the scientists and clinicians involved. Protocols should be carefully designed in order to obtain as much information as possible from the pilot studies. This will involve recording all vital signs before, during, and after administration and full biochemical

TABLE 4.8. Absorbed Radiation Doses from Selected Antibody Preparations (mGy MBq^{-1})

Immunoradiopharmaceutical

Organs	I-131-OC125 F(ab$'$)$_2$ (IMACIS 2) International CIS	In-111-OC125 F(ab$'$)$_2$ (INDIMACIS) International CIS	Tc-99m-250/183 (GRANULOZYT) Behringwerke	Tc-99m-431/26 (ANTI-CEA) Behringwerke	In-111-C46 (ANTI-CEA) Amersham	In-P256Fab$'$ (PLATELET SPECIFIC) Amersham	I-123MAB-A47 (GRANULOSZINT) Mallinckrodt
Whole body	0.2	0.11	0.010	0.014	0.6	0.75	0.015
Liver	1.3	0.75	0.011	0.008	1.0	0.71	0.069
Lungs	—	—	0.008	—	—	0.14	0.013
Spleen	—	0.59	0.008	—	—	9.68	0.087
Kidneys	—	0.49	0.022	0.014	2.3	0.68	0.017
Gonads	0.2	—	0.006	—	0.7	0.08	0.014
Bone marrow	—	—	0.016	0.006	—	0.14	0.078
Thyroid	148.0[a]	—	—	—	—	0.03[a]	0.008
Stomach	—	—	—	—	—	—	0.014

[a] Data obtained without thyroid blocking agent.

TABLE 4.9. Basic Parameters for Imaging Studies With Radiolabelled Monoclonal Antibodies[a]

	131-I	123-I	111-In	99mTc
Radiopharmaceutical	100 µg—1 mg (or greater) monoclonal antibody			
Radionuclide	131-I	123-I	111-In	99mTc
Activity administered	80 MBq (2mCi) (100 MBq (3 mCi) 99Tc-HSA 100 MBq (3 mCi) 99mTc for background subtraction)	80 MBq (2mCi)	80 MBq (2 mCi)	400 MBq (10 mCi)
Radiation dose				
Effective dose equivalent	10 mSv (1000 mrem)	6 mSv (600 mrem)	10 mSv (1000 mrem)	4 mSv (400 mrem)
Organ dose	Thyroid 104 mGy (10400 mrad) Liver 20–60 mGy (2000–6000 mrad)	Thyroid 50 MBq (500 mrad) Liver 10–20 mGy (1000–2000 mrad)	Liver 70–100 mGy (7000–10000 mrad) Kidneys 70–100 mGy (7000–10000 mrad)	Liver 10–20 mGy (1000–2000 mrad) Kidneys 14 mGy (1400 mrad)
Patient preparation	Oral sodium iodide 60 mg for 7 days	Oral sodium iodide 60 mg for 3 days	Oral laxatives and bowel preparation may be necessary	
Collimator	High energy, parallel hole	Low energy parallel hole	Medium energy, parallel hole	Low energy, parallel hole
Images acquired	Anterior and posterior images as required			
	200 k counts	600 k counts	600 k counts	600 k counts
	3–7 days	4–24 hours	4–72 hours	4–18 hours
SPECT		64 × 20 second increments in 360° rotation. Useful in brain, thorax, abdomen, and pelvis.		

[a] Approximate figures given. Organ doses are based on a 80 MBq dose of intact antibody but will depend upon the antibody and fragments used and may vary with repeat administrations. For example, the liver dose will be higher if HAMA is present.

and haematological sampling before and after administration of the antibody. In fact, the evaluation of the images themselves is comparatively simple when compared to the analysis of any variations in clinical parameters during clinical trials.

One of the most important characteristics of a particular antibody is its target to non-target (T:NT) uptake. Whilst quantification of uptake may be obtained from gamma camera images, this only provides a measure of the image contrast, and although uptake in the lesion or tumour may be clearly visible, selection of a normal area of tissue may be particularly difficult. In the case of tumour-associated antibodies, the tumour to normal tissue uptake may be measured directly by the assay of radioactivity in resected tumour and normal tissues. If the tissue specimens are weighed and assayed for radioactivity, the results may then be expressed as a count rate per gram of tissue and the T:NT calculated accordingly. This information may be obtained without any additional inconvenience to patients who are referred for curative surgery, although it is easier to obtain from patients with primary tumours, since recurrent disease and metastases are not always treated by surgery. Measurement of the uptake of a radiolabelled antibody in this way does not, however, confirm the specificity of an antibody for the particular lesion involved. The only true measure is obtained following the simultaneous assay of the uptake of the radiolabelled antibody and an irrelevant immunoglobulin of the same isotype. In this way a localisation index may be obtained. This does present additional problems of the preparation and administration of a further immunological product to the patient. Furthermore, the logistics of choosing a second radiolabel suitable for clinical administration add to the burden of assessing any

particular antibody. In the case of the antibody 791T/36 the authors were involved in the simultaneous administration of I-131-labelled antibody and I-123-labelled IgG2b in order to determine this information. However, this was only measured in a single patient (Armitage et al., 1984).

In the case of antibodies directed against antigens associated with benign conditions, the assay of T:NT uptake in tissue samples is not always possible. With antibodies directed against blood cells, characterisation of the product may be carried out by the assay of the cellular fractions recovered in a blood sample taken following administration of the antibody. Such information is also of value in the case of tumour-associated antibodies to check for any cross reactivity with cellular components and products in the circulation (Pimm et al., 1985).

In some instances the intravenous administration of antibody has resulted in unexpected effects. Dillman et al. (1984) reported the suppression of circulating granulocytes following administration of anti-CEA antibody. This highlights the necessity for assessing the full range of interactions which could compromise the patient participating in the trial, and, of course, such adverse reactions would result in an immediate cessation of the clinical administration of a particular antibody.

ANTIBODY CHARACTERISTICS

It is now common to find a number of antibodies produced by different institutions which appear to react with the same antigen, or perhaps different epitopes of the same antigen. For example, a number of antibodies directed against CEA have been produced and used for both experimental and clinical imaging. Given that some of the epitopes of CEA are also expressed on normal cross-reacting antigen (NCA), some anti-CEA antibodies will be more suitable as radiopharmaceuticals than others. The diverse physicochemical properties of anti-CEA antibodies indicates that *in vitro* studies and tumour imaging in mice with tumour xenografts are not fully capable of indicating the suitability of an antibody for tumour imaging (Pimm et al., 1987).

Despite all the available methods for pre-clinical testing, the final characteristics of any particular antibody, when incorporated into a radiopharmaceutical, will not be appreciated until radiolabelling studies and clinical imaging has been undertaken. In Nottingham three murine anti-CEA monoclonal antibodies designated 161, 198 (both IgG1) and 228 (IgG2a) were produced by standard hybridoma techniques. Whilst 228 antibody appeared to be specific for CEA, *in vitro* studies showed 161 and 198 to cross react with NCA. Following reaction with DTPA anhydride, the efficiency of chelation of In-111 varied with mean values of 30%, 52% and 62%, respectively, and gel filtration chromatography demonstrated radiolabel to be predominantly coincident with IgG. *In vivo* studies in mice showed that In-111 was excreted at virtually the same rate with half-times of the order of 12 days. Imaging of tumour xenografts expressing CEA was successfully achieved with all antibodies resulting in T:NT image contrast of up to 5:1. However, the imaging capabilities of these three antibodies in patients with colorectal cancer was markedly different (Fig. 4.6). The main characteristic of the images of six patients injected with In-111-161 antibody was that of high liver uptake, and only one out of six tumours was detected from the images. With In-111-198 antibody intense uptake of tracer was observed throughout the bone

marrow, and only 1 of 5 tumours was visualised. The images of patients injected with 228 antibody showed intermediate liver and bone marrow uptake, and four of six tumours were detected. These studies illustrate the diverse nature and unexpected properties of antibodies which are ultimately incorporated into radiopharmaceuticals for imaging.

INTERPRETATION OF ANTIBODY IMAGES

As with any radionuclide imaging investigation, the interpretation of the images is a skill which must be learnt by experience. This experience is based on recognition of the abnormal from the normal. The early images that were obtained from patients injected with radiolabelled antibodies were extremely difficult to understand. This was mainly due to technical factors, in particular the use of radionuclides with poor physical characteristics, such as I-131, and the use of antibodies with low target to non-target uptake. As a result, the image enhancement procedures that were adopted could lead to errors in diagnosis. The main false-positive sites in subtraction images using I-131-labelled antibodies are described in Chapter 5, this volume.

The development of reliable procedures for radiolabelling antibodies with I-123, In-111, and Tc-99m have enabled images to be recorded in the same way as with any other radiopharmaceutical. Given the present state of the art, images may be recorded directly onto nuclear medicine film without the need for computer manipulation. In this way antibody imaging has developed to the level of a routine imaging procedure. Since the images primarily convey physiological information rather than anatomical information, it is necessary to have a series of views recorded over

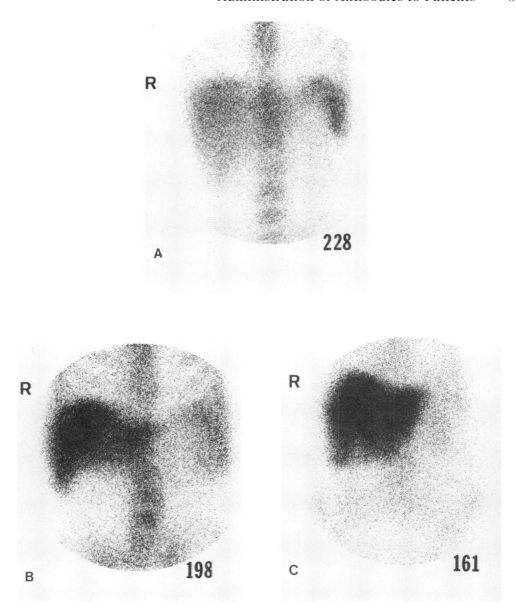

Fig. 4.6. Typical examples of images obtained using 3 different anti-CEA antibodies, showing anterior views of the upper abdomen. **A:** In-111-228 showing intermediate liver and bone marrow activity. **B:** In-111-198 showing high bone marrow and liver uptake. **C:** In-161 showing intense liver activity (not due to HAMA). 198 and 161 antibody were known to cross-react with NCA. (From the authors' unpublished studies.)

a set time period. The timing of the images will depend upon the nature of the immunoradiopharmaceutical, i.e., intact antibody or fragments and, of course, the physical half-life of the radiolabel. The images obtained with I-123 (and I-131) may show uptake in the thyroid gland (despite the administration of a blocking agent), gastric mucosa, and the urinary tract. With radiometals such as In-111 and Tc-99m, the tracer is rapidly taken up by the reticuloendothelial system, and therefore activity is seen throughout the liver, spleen, and bone marrow. Whilst high levels of liver uptake do prevent the visualisation of small liver metastases, large metastases can be seen as cold areas on early blood pool views with some "in-filling" on the latter views recorded at 48–72 hours. With some Tc-99m antibodies, metastases may be visualised as areas of increased uptake above the liver activity. If the patient has had a previous dose of antibody and HAMA is present, the liver uptake is likely to be more intense following a subsequent administration.

Bone marrow activity provides an anatomical landmark for identifying the position of abnormal sites of uptake and is a particularly useful aid for identifying sites of uptake using emission computed tomography. Occasionally activity may present in the kidneys and urinary bladder, depending upon the antibody and radiolabel used and the condition of the patient. This may be seen on the early blood pool images and occasionally on the delayed images. However, it is unusual to see activity at these sites on the delayed views if it is not present on the blood pool views. Fairly intense adrenal uptake may be frequently seen, and testicular uptake is also frequently observed using some In-111-labelled antibodies.

The blood pool views provide an indication of the presence of any abnormality in the great vessels, particularly in the chest, pelvis, and limbs. Any large cystic areas may be seen as areas of reduced uptake on the blood pool views. Ascites also initially shows up as reduced areas of activity, which may often appear as bands or a "halo" around organs. On the delayed views simple cystic areas generally remain as areas of reduced uptake and have a smooth outline, whereas malignant ascites will generally take up activity as shown by the assay of radioactivity in cystic and ascitic fluid. Abnormal "hot" uptake within a cystic area provides an indication of possible malignancy.

A particular problem with In-111-labelled antibodies has been the presence of tracer within both the small and large bowel. This may be easy to visualise, for example, in the ascending, transverse, and descending colon, in which case it is not usually a problem, but occasionally this may prevent a definite diagnosis being made. Repeat imaging may be necessary to assess whether there is any movement of tracer along the bowel. With a good antibody, positive tumour uptake is often more intense than the activity in the bowel; however, if tumour uptake is not clear-cut, bowel uptake could result in a false-positive diagnosis.

In some cases emission tomography is useful for a clearer identification of the sites of activity within the abdomen and pelvis. The transaxial views provide a means for visualising the depth of sites of activity within the abdomen and help in the identification of bowel activity. Emission tomography should be used whenever possible in these investigations to obtain the most accurate diagnosis.

REFERENCES AND FURTHER READING

Armitage, N.C., Perkins, A.C., Pimm, M.V., Farrands, P.A., Baldwin, R.W., and Hardcastle, J.D. (1984):

The localisation of an anti-tumour monoclonal antibody (791T/36) in gastrointestinal tumours. Br. J. Surg. 71:407–412.

Bosslet, K., Streinstraser, A., Schwarz, A., Harthus, H.P., Lubenm, G., Kuhlmann, L., Sedlacek, H.H. (1988): Quantitative considerations supporting the irrelevance of circulating serum CEA for the immunoscintigraphic visualisation of CEA expressing carcinoma. Eur. J. Nucl. Med. 14:523–528.

Britton, K.E., Buraggi, G.L., Bares, R., Bischof-Delaloye, A., Buell, U., Emrich, D., and Granowska, M. (1989): A brief guide to the practice of radioimmunoscintigraphy and radioimmunotherapy in cancer. Int. J. Biol. Markers 4:106–118.

Burragi, G.L., Callegaro, L., Mariani, G., Turrin, A., Cascinelli, N., Attili, A., Bombardieri, E., Terno, G., Plassio, G., Dovis, M., Mazzuca, N., Nacali, P.G., Scassellati, G.A., Rose, U., Ferrone, S. (1985): Imaging with I-131 labeled monoclonal antibodies to a high molecular weight melanoma associated antigen in patients with melanoma: Efficacy of whole immunoglobulin and its F(ab')$_2$ fragments. Cancer Res. 45:3378–3387.

Carrasquillo, J.A., Sugarbaker, P., Colcher, D., Reynolds, J.C., Esterban, J., Bryant, G., Keenan, A.M., Perentesis, P., Yokoyama, K., Simpson, D.E., Ferroni, P., Farkas, R., Schlom, J., Larson, S.M. (1988): Radioimmunoscintigraphy of colon cancer with iodine-131-labeled B72.3 monoclonal antibody. J. Nucl. Med. 29:0122–1030.

Centre for Drugs and Biologics, U.S. Food and Drug Administration (1987): Points to consider in the manufacture and testing of monoclonal antibody products for human use. Washington, D.C.: U.S. Government Printing Office.

Colcher, D., Esterban, J.M., Carrasquillo, J.A., Sugarbaker, P., Reynolds, J.C., Bryant, G., Larson, S.M., Schlom, J. (1987): Quantitative analyses of selective radiolabeled monoclonal antibody localization in metastatic lesions of colorectal cancer patients. Cancer Res. 47:1185–1189.

Commission of the European Communities (1989): Guidelines on radiopharmaceuticals based on monoclonal antibodies. In: Ad Hoc Working Party on Biotechnology/Pharmacy: Notes for Guidance. Luxembourg: Office for Official Publications of the European Communities.

Dillman, R.O., Beauregard, J., Sobol, R.E., Royston, I., Bartholomew, R.M., Hagan, P.S., Halpern, S.E. (1984): Lack of radioimmunodetection and complications associated with monoclonal anticarcinoembryonic antigen antibody cross reactivity with an antigen on circulating cells. Cancer Res. 44: 2213–2218.

Eger, R.R., Covell, D.G., Carrasquillo, J.A., Abrams, P.G., Foon, K.A., Reynolds, J.C., Schroff, R.W., Morgan, A.C., Larson, S.M., Weinstein, J.N. (1987): Kinetic model for biodistribution of an In-111 labeled monoclonal antibody in humans. Cancer Res. 47:3328–3336.

Hnatowich, D.J., Griffen, T.W., Kosciuczyk, C., Rusckowski, M., Childs, R.L., Mattis, J.A., Shealy,

D., Doherty, P.W. (1985): Pharmacokinetics of an indium-111 labeled monoclonal antibody in cancer patients. J. Nucl. Med. 26:849–858.

Hnatowich, D.J., Gionet, M., Rusckowski, M., Siebecker, D.A., Roche, J., Shealy, D., Mattis, J.A., Wilson, J., McGann, J., Hunter, R.E., Griffin, T., Doherty, P.W. (1987): Pharmacokinetics of In-111 labeled OC-125 antibody in cancer patients compared with the 19-9 antibody. Cancer Res. 47:6111–6117.

International Commission on Radiological Protection (1987): Protection of the patient in nuclear medicine (ICRP publication 52). Ann. ICRP 17:No. 4.

International Commission on Radiological Protection (1987): Radiation dose to patients from pharmaceuticals (ICRP Publication 53), Ann. ICRP 18:No. 1–4.

Lamki, L.M., Murray, J.L., Rosenblum, M.G., Patt, Y.Z., Babaian, R., Unger, M.W. (1988): Effect of unlabelled monoclonal antibody (MoAb) on biodistribution of indium-111 labelled (MoAb). Nucl. Med. Commun. 9:553–564.

Mach, J-P., Buchegger, F., Forni, M., Ritschard, J., Berche, C., Lumbroso, J-D., Schreyer, M., Girardet, C., Accolla, R.S., Carrel, S. (1981): Use of radiolabelled monoclonal anti-CEA antibody for the detection of human carcinomas by external photoscanning and tomoscintigraphy. Immunol. Today 2:239–249.

Malamitsi, J., Skarlos, D., Fotious, S., Papakostas, P., Aravantinos, G., Vassilarou, D., Taylor-Papadimitriou, J., Koutoulidis, K., Hooker, G., Snook, D., Epenetos, A.A. (1988): Intracavity use of two radiolabeled tumor associated monoclonal antibodies. J. Nucl. Med. 29:1915–1920.

Medical Internal Radiation Dose Committee (1975): Pamphlet 11. Society of Nuclear Medicine, 404 Church Avenue, Suite 15, Maryville, TN 37801, USA.

Murray, J.L., Rosenblum, M.G., Sobol, R.E., Bartholomew, R.M., Plager, C.E., Haynie, T.P., Jahns, M.F., Glenn, H.J., Lamki, L., Benjamin, R.S., Papadopoulos, N., Boddie, A.W., Frincke, J.M., David, G.S., Carlo, D.J., Hersh, E.M. (1985): Radioimmunoimaging in malignant melanoma with In-111 labeled monoclonal antibody 96.5. Cancer Res. 45:2376–2381.

Murray, J.L., Lamki, L.M., Shanken, L.J., Blake, M.E., Plager, C.E., Benjamin, R.S., Schweighardt, S., Unger, M.W., Rosenblum, M.G. (1988): Immunospecific saturable clearance mechanism for indium-111-labeled anti-melanoma monoclonal antibody 96.5 in humans. Cancer Res. 48:4417–4422.

Perkins, A.C., Pimm, M.V. (1985): Differences in tumour and normal tissue concentrations of Iodine and Indium-labelled monoclonal antibody. I. The effect on image contrast in clinical studies. Eur. J. Nucl. Med. 11:295–299.

Perkins, A.C., Pimm, M.V., Gie, C., Marksmans, R.A., Symonds, E.M., Baldwin, R.W. (1989): Intraperitoneal I-131 and In-111-791T/36 monoclonal antibody imaging in recurrent ovarian cancer: Imaging and biodistribution. Nucl. Med. Commun. 10: 577–584.

Pimm, M.V., Perkins, A.C., Armitage, N.C., Baldwin, R.W. (1985): The characteristics of blood-borne radiolabels and the effect of anti-mouse IgG antibodies on localization of radiolabeled monoclonal antibody in cancer patients. J. Nucl. Med. 26: 1011–1023.

Pimm, M.V., Perkins, A.C., Baldwin, R.W. (1985): Differences in tumour and normal tissue concentrations of Iodine and Indium-labelled monoclonal antibody. II. Biodistribution studies in mice with human tumour xenografts. Eur. J. Nucl. Med. 11:300–304.

Pimm, M.V., Perkins, A.C., Baldwin, R.W. (1987): Diverse characteristics of In-111-labelled and anti-CEA monoclonal antibodies for tumour immunoscintigraphy: Radiolabelling, biodistribution and imaging studies in mice with human tumour xenografts. Eur. J. Nucl. Med. 12:515–521.

Powell, M.C., Perkins, A.C., Pimm, M.V., Al, Jetaily, M., Wastie, M.L., Durrant, L., Baldwin, R.W., Symonds, E.M. (1987): Diagnostic imaging of gynecological tumors with the monoclonal antibody 791T/36. Am. J. Obstet. Gynecol. 157:28–34.

Roedler, V., Lechel, U. (1988): Administered activity and dose for immunoscintigraphy. Eur. J. Nucl. Med. 14:C6 (abstract).

Rosenblum, M.G., Murray, J.L., Haynie, T.P., Glenn, H.J., Jahns, M.F., Benjamin, R.S., Frinke, J.M., Carlo, D.J., Hersh, E.M. (1985): Pharmacokinetics of indium-111-labeled anti-p67 monoclonal antibody in patients with metastatic melanoma. Cancer Res. 45:2382–2386.

Shepherd, P.S., Lazarus, C.R., Mistry, R.D., Maisey, M.N. (1985): Detection of thyroid tumours using monoclonal I-123 anti-human thyroglobulin antibody. Eur. J. Nucl. Med. 10:291–295.

Thomas, G.D., Chappell, M.J., Dykes, P.W., Ramsden, D.B., Godfrey, K.R., Ellis, J.R.M., Bradwell, A.R. (1989): Effect of dose, molecular size, affinity and protein binding on tumour uptake of antibody or ligand: A biomathematical model. Cancer Res. 49:3290–3296.

Ward, B.G., Mather, S.J., Hawkins, L.R., Crowther, M.E., Shepherd, J.H., Granowska, M., Britton, K.E., Slevin, M.L. (1987): Localization of radioiodine conjugated to the monoclonal antibody HMFG2 in human ovarian carcinoma: Assessment of intravenous and intraperitoneal routes of administration. Cancer Res. 47:4719–4723.

Wochner, R.D., Adatepe, M., Van Amberg, A., Potchen, E.J. (1970): A new method for estimation of plasma volume with the use of the distribution space of indium-113m-transferrin. J. Lab. Clin. Med. 75:711–720.

5 Imaging Techniques

INTRODUCTION

The detection of pathology using radiolabelled antibodies is dependent upon both the *in vivo* biodistribution of the immunoradiopharmaceutical and the physical characteristics of the radionuclide and the imaging system. The main criticism of immunoscintigraphy with antibodies that have previously been available has been the relatively poor lesion uptake compared to that in surrounding tissues. Although this is partly related to the relative antigen expression between normal and abnormal sites, it is also related to the choice of radionuclide and the efficiency of photon detection during the imaging procedure. A list of the main factors affecting the image quality is given in Table 5.1. The quality of the final image therefore is affected by advances in many varied specialities ranging from immunology and biotechnology through to chemistry, physics, and computing. It is probably the combination of these factors which make the technique of immunoscintigraphy so unique and in this way attracts the skills of many workers from throughout these varied disciplines.

Factors affecting the choice of antibody and radiolabel for imaging have been discussed in Chapters 1 and 2, this volume. In this chapter a description of the imaging procedures is given together with details of the various image processing techniques that have been applied for lesion detection from antibody images. Given that the antibodies that are currently available are far from perfect, image processing manoeuvres have been applied to overcome their poor abilities for localisation. The majority of earlier studies were carried out using I-131 as the radiolabel, mainly due to the ease of protein iodination as compared with radiolabelling using other more suitable radiolabels for scintigraphy. The use of I-131 as the radiolabel placed immediate constraints on the accuracy of lesion detection. Its high energy of gamma emission results in poor image resolution and lower detection efficiency with correspondingly low count rates per unit dose. Clearly the use of lower energy radiolabels such as Tc-99m, which is more suitable for modern gamma cameras, will result in improvements in image quality, thereby re-

TABLE 5.1. Factors Affecting Lesion Detection by Immunoscintigraphy

Choice of antibody

  Antigenic determinants
  Species of origin
  Immunoglobulin isotype
  Fragmentation of antibody molecule
  Bioengineering variables

Choice of radiolabel

  Energy of photon emission
  Physical half-life
  Periodic group (i.e., metal or halide)
  Chemical conjugation
  Patient dosimetry

Imaging technique

  Planar imaging
  Whole body scanning
  Emission tomography

Image processing

  Thresholding
  Saturation
  Smoothing
  Filtration
  Reconstruction
  Statistical analysis
  Dynamic analysis and probability mapping

Background subtraction

  Dual radionuclide subtraction
  Subtraction of early from late images
  Administration of second antibody

Image recording and interpretation

  Observer experience
  Transparent film display
  TV display

ducing the need for complicated image analysis. In addition, the continued advances in the design and performance of imaging equipment have resulted in im-

provements in image quality, adding to the clinical value of the technique.

THE IMAGING PROBLEM

As with any scintigraphic image, the information presented to the observer usually consists of a two-dimensional projection of a three-dimensional distribution of the radionuclide within the patient. The pulses generated by the gamma camera contain information on the spatial distribution of events (x and y coordinates) and a signal of their acceptance (z) following energy discrimination. Following digitisation by computer, the events are registered in a matrix of cells commonly 64×64, 128×128 or 256×256 wide. Image digitisation permits both the qualitative and quantitative extraction of data. However, because the image is made up of a recorded number of counts, the finite statistics of the detected events affect the final contrast resolution above the background noise. Visualisation of the lesion is generally measured in terms of image contrast (IC), which may be defined as

$$IC = \frac{Ct - Cnt}{Cnt},$$

where Ct = the target count rate and Cnt = the non-target count rate. The detection of a lesion taking up radiolabelled antibody in an image is essentially a problem of poor signal-to-noise levels; hence the application of image processing routines to extract the relevant data from the image.

The theoretical limits of detection relative to the size and depths of lesions have been investigated by a number of workers. Lakshmanan et al. (1978) carried out studies in phantoms to simulate the detection of abnormalities during brain imaging using Tc-99m-pertechnetate and concluded that an abnormality in the form of a 8 mm diameter cylinder was the smallest lesion detectable at a concentration ratio of 22.5:1. Rockoff et al. (1980) considered the immunodetection of tumours using the net difference in the two-dimensional image count rates between the effective signal area (in this case tumour) and an equivalent background area as the detection criterion. They concluded that the detection of a 1 cm square lesion at depth of about 5 cm required a target to non-target ratio (T:NT) of over 5:1, although this would vary with background count rates. This approach was, however, rather simplistic, as it only considered the projected area of the signal and failed to account for the tumour volume. A more rigorous approach to modelling the detection of tumours using radiolabelled antibody was carried out by Bradwell et al. (1985). This approach was based on that of Rockoff but examined a much wider range of parameters affecting lesion detection. The factors affecting the immunodetection of tumours were defined mathematically and combined in the form of equations which could be solved to predict the outcome for tumour detection and therapy. The model was based on 11 parameters which could be defined within the patient and the imaging equipment. These are given in Table 5.2. This model was developed on the concept that optimum detection was achieved using the process of dual radionuclide image subtraction, which is described subsequently. However, it did indicate that the use of a subtraction radionuclide did increase the image noise, and this degraded the final image quality. The results showed that a tumour of 5 mm diameter at a depth of 5 cm within the patient would require a T:NT uptake ratio of 20:1.

The calculations indicated that the two most important factors affecting tumour detection were those of T:NT ratio and the

TABLE 5.2. Parameters Used
for the Mathematical Modelling
of Immunoscintigraphy
(adapted from Bradwell et al.,1985)

1. Tumour area (mm)
2. Tumour depth (mm)
3. Body depth (mm)
4. Signal-to-noise ratio
5. Lesion to normal tissue uptake ratio
6. Count rate from radiolabelled antibody/ square centimetre
7. Count rate from subtraction radionuclide/ square centimetre
8. Gamma ray attenuation
9. Gamma camera resolution (FWHM in millimetres)
10. Collimator hole diameter (mm)
11. Collimator hole depth (mm)

absolute count rate of the administered radiolabelled antibody. These results came as no surprise, since the fundamental limitations of antibodies which were available at that time were those of poor specificity for the target tissues and the use of I-131 which is poorly suited for use with modern gamma cameras. It was for these very reasons that image enhancement techniques were being applied in order to improve lesion detection.

IMAGE COUNTS AND COUNT RATES

The importance of recorded image counts can not be overemphasised, since as in any radionuclide imaging procedure using the gamma camera, superior image quality results from increased acquired counts. The stochastic nature of radioactive decay results in statistical noise which may be assumed to have a Poissonian distribution. The background noise in the image primarily originates from electronic noise in the imaging equipment and cosmic radiation and other naturally occurring radioactivity in the region of the detector. With most radiopharmaceuticals the background noise may be removed by thresholding the lower level of image display (see below).

As the object of the imaging process is to determine whether there is any abnormality in the biodistribution of the administered imaging agent, it is important that the information within the image is of the highest quality. This ultimately rests in the numerical statistics of the detected events. Thus the number and distribution of the detected events affect the confidence with which the final diagnosis may be made. The count rate available for imaging is dependent on the amount of radionuclide administered, the energy of its gamma emission, and its detection efficiency by the scintillation crystal-photomultiplier assembly. The amount of radioactivity which may be administered is limited for reasons of patient dosimetry. In general terms the amount of radioactivity administered will be the minimum necessary for obtaining the required result. This amount will be a balance weighing the potential benefit from the results of the investigation against the possible harm from the administered dose of radiation. Clearly the absolute amount of radioactivity administered may vary depending upon the clinical condition being investigated. It would be unethical to administer large amounts of radioactivity to patients being investigated with benign conditions, but large doses of radioactivity may be insignificant in patients who are also undergoing radiotherapy for malignancy. The doses of radioactivity administered for routine clinical use and research purposes are generally restricted by Hospital Ethical Committees and by the Departments of Health in the various countries of Europe and in the United States.

Radionuclide images consist of a number of events detected over a period of time. The choice of radionuclide for antibody radiolabelling clearly affects the quality of the final image from a point of view of both image resolution and count rate. For example, in the authors' experience, when imaging patients using I-131-labelled antibody, imaging 3 to 5 days after administration often took over 30 minutes per view. This may not always be possible in busy nuclear medicine departments.

It has clearly been the introduction of radiolabels such as In-111, I-123, and Tc-99m with lower energies, finer resolution, and a corresponding increase in detection efficiency per unit of dose that has resulted in the improvements in image quality that have recently been observed. In general terms, following a dose of 80–120 MBq of one of these radionuclides satisfactory planar images may be obtained by the acquisition of 600–800 k counts over a 40 cm field of view in a time period of about 5 minutes. It follows also that these radionuclides will provide count rates sufficient for antibody emission tomography to be completed within relatively short time periods for data collection, i.e., 30 to 60 minutes (see below).

Image Display

The detection of a lesion by immunoscintigraphy, a process of distinguishing abnormal from normal distribution, is a subjective process which ultimately depends upon observer experience. Commonly this process is carried out in a dark-adapted environment using illuminated single emulsion transparent film on which the detected counts are displayed as differing levels of grey. Detection of a lesion thus depends upon the recognition of significant change in contrast between the normal and abnormal regions. In many ways the transparent film is not the best medium for image viewing since the dynamic range of the film is non-linear and distortion of the displayed information may occur. However, satisfactory results are now routinely obtained with transparent film and using antibodies radiolabelled with Tc-99m, I-123, and In-111. In this way immunoscintigraphy may be carried out in the same manner as any other standard radionuclide imaging procedure.

The use of digital images generated by computers and displayed on TV systems provides a means for both the subjective and quantitative evaluation of image data. The computer may be used for a range of image processing routines for image enhancement as well as for the statistical analysis of image data. Such displays are essential for the manipulation and evaluation of tomographic images.

IMAGE ENHANCEMENT
Image Display Windowing

Given that many immunoradiopharmaceuticals have poor specificity for target lesions, the difference in the recorded counts for individual image pixels representing normal and abnormal areas may be small compared to the total number of counts in the image. Using the full range of display levels, such differences may not be apparent. Contrast enhancement may be achieved by windowing the display in a digital image to show the pixels having values within a particular range of interest. The pixels with the lowest count rates may be thresholded, by displaying only those pixels with counts above a minimum level, and the pixels with the highest count rate may be saturated, by setting a maximum level for the display. Such manipulations may be performed rapidly on all nuclear

medicine computer systems and will often lead to an increase in the confidence with which a lesion may be identified. In immunoscintigraphy, alteration of the display levels in this way is particularly useful where there are other sites of radionuclide concentration in the image. This has been found useful in identification of lesions in the lower abdomen and pelvis, using iodinated antibody in the presence of large amounts of free radioiodide in the urinary bladder, and for the localisations of lesions in the upper abdomen and thorax, using In-111-labelled antibody, which concentrates in high amounts in the liver.

Image Arithmetic

The values of the individual pixels within the image may be altered by arithmetic operations such as addition, subtraction, multiplication, and division. The use of image processing techniques is now commonplace within nuclear medicine, and some procedures have been successfully applied to antibody images to increase the detection rates of lesions (mainly tumours). One technique which has been subject to a great deal of attention is image subtraction using a background image of a non-specific tracer. This was first applied to antibody imaging by DeLand et al. (1980), and it had a dramatic effect on the detection rate of tumours using the I-131-labelled antibodies that were available at that time. The image subtraction process is described in detail subsequently.

The particular image processing routine to be applied generally depends upon the information required from the image, and some prior knowledge of the subject intensity distribution is usually assumed (Goris and Briandet, 1983). Processing routines are usually interactive with the operator and may be used to improve the subjective interpretation of the images. Quantitative data from the images will be affected to an extent depending upon the applied processing routine. In general, image processing is complicated by the inverse relationship between image noise and image resolution. For example, noise reduction necessitates some form of averaging the image information, and this impairs resolution. Improving the resolution adds higher frequency information, thus increasing the image noise. In general, the processing applications which are suitable for immunoscintigraphy are image smoothing, filtering, and image refocussing.

Statistical variations in antibody images will be especially high in situations where the total number of collected counts are low. Such variations may be smoothed by spatial averaging. This may be achieved by taking an arithmetic average of the count rates in surrounding pixels or by averaging with a weighted filter (for example, a pseudo-Gaussian 9-point weighted filter). The use of such a smoothing filter is particularly suitable for the low count density images obtained with I-131-labelled antibody. Weighted filters are also employed in the filtered back projection process used for the reconstruction of SPECT images.

Image refocussing methods, such as deconvolution, are mathematical techniques which increase the spatial frequency components in the image which are inevitably lost by the image acquisition process. The presence of noise in the system places major constraints on these procedures and the algorithms employed are often cumbersome, utilising a great deal of computer time.

Feature Detection

A large number of image processing techniques involve the extraction of a required component of image information. The aim in this case is to maximise the required signal or feature at the expense of the remainder of the information. Image processing techniques of this kind have been taken from other non-medical realms of scientific exploration, astronomy in particular. Methods of feature detection commonly involve the use of edge detection algorithms to highlight a particular contour level. Fairweather et al. (1983) described a procedure for the automatic processing of antibody images, which involved three main steps. Firstly, dual radionuclide subtraction was performed to remove the non-target activity, then image noise was removed using a Wiener filter, and finally a non-linear deconvolution (maximum entropy) technique was applied and the final image expressed in contour plots in units of standard deviation. A similar standardised processing technique for use in immunoscintigraphy has been proposed by Liehn et al. (1987). This involves the following three main stages of processing: 1) geometric image registration, 2) image normalisation and 3) production of an image of significant differences. These processes are described subsequently.

In general, the use of automatic processing techniques to avoid observer bias have not been widely adopted because of the complicated nature of the images and the computer time necessary to run these routines. The main problem with these particular approaches were the detection of false-positive areas of uptake due to the non-specific uptake of labelled antibody or as a result of the image subtraction and processing procedures used.

BACKGROUND SUBTRACTION
Dual Radionuclide
Image Subtraction

Dual radionuclide image subtraction has been used in nuclear medicine to overcome the poor localising properties of some radiopharmaceuticals. In instances where the difference in the target and background concentrations is not as high as desirable, image enhancement of the target tissues may be achieved by removing the unwanted background counts from the surrounding tissues using a second radionuclide to simulate the non-target activity. This was first described by Kaplan et al. (1966) for imaging the pancreas using Se-75-selenomethionine, which concentrates in both the pancreas and liver. Following the simultaneous administration of Tc-99m sulphur colloid, or colloidal Au-198, the resulting liver image was subtracted to leave the activity within the pancreas. Similarly the uptake of Ga-67 by abscesses may be masked by activity in surrounding tissues. The background activity from liver, spleen, and lungs was removed using Tc-99m-sulphur colloid and Tc-99m-human serum albumin (Beihn et al., 1974). Skretting et al. (1978) reported the use of a triple radionuclide subtraction technique. Iodine-131-labelled toluidine blue was used to localise enlarged parathyroid glands, and corrections were applied for the circulating radioiodine and for that trapped by the thyroid, using In-113m-labelled transferrin and Tc-99m-pertechnetate, respectively.

The use of dual radionuclide image subtraction to overcome poor image contrast in the immunoscintigraphy of tumours was first described by DeLand et al. (1980). Since this time, background subtraction has received much attention by workers in immunoscintigraphy, and therefore it will be described in detail here. The majority of human studies reported during the late 1970s and early 1980s using I-131-labelled antibodies associated with tumour antigens showed that tumour uptake of antibody was low (T:NT uptake ratio of about 2:1). The main feature of these studies was

the large proportion of the administered dose remaining in the circulation, reducing the image contrast between the tumour and non-tumour tissues. Using a second tracer to simulate the non-target activity (usually Tc-99m), background subtraction could be performed to enhance the detection of uptake within the tumour tissues. During the early 1980s a large number of published clinical studies reported the use of external imaging of antibody localisation using I-131-labelled antibodies with Tc-99m-blood pool subtraction (Goldenberg et al., 1978, 1980; Goldenberg and DeLand, 1982; Farrands et al., 1982; Begent et al., 1983). The use of the subtraction technique increased the tumour to background image contrast by a factor of two, raising the sensitivity of the technique to above 70%.

The physical nature of the radiopharmaceutical and its gamma emissions, together with the geometrical relationship between the patient and the detector, will limit the ability to achieve an accurate representation of the distribution of the radiopharmaceutical *in vivo*. The image of the events registered by the detector consist of a two-dimensional array of radioactivity distributed in three dimensions within the patient. A mathematical description of this was first described by DeLand et al. (1980) and later expanded by Liehn (1988). A simple two-compartmental model may be used to illustrate the basic process of subtraction (Fig. 5.1). Because of the relatively poor specificity of the target radiopharmaceutical, it concentrates in both the target and non-target tissues (recorded as image matrix A). The non-target radiopharmaceutical should concentrate in the non-target tissues only (recorded as matrix B). Subtraction of the non-target distribution should leave the target concentration (matrix C), even if the original count rate density in T and NT were constant. If the sub-

A.

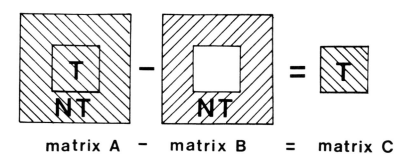

matrix A   –   matrix B   =   matrix C

B.

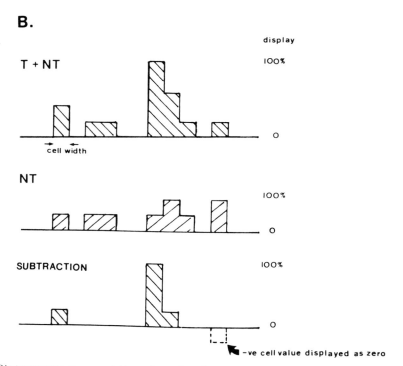

Fig. 5.1. **A:** Diagrammatic representation of matrix subtraction using a simple two compartment model. **B:** Diagrammatic representation of a line (n) of pixels in a digital image containing target and non-target information. Subtraction of line (n) of the non-target image leaves the target information (scaled to 100%).

traction process is achieved perfectly, the non-target counts are completely removed and the T:NT uptake becomes infinite. However, this is never achieved in practice because it is impossible to achieve a perfect non-target image and because of statistical variations and noise in the two images. In practice this process is much more complicated than as described above. Firstly, the images must be recorded with the patient in exactly the same position (image congruence). This point is satisfied if simultaneous dual radionuclide acquisition is performed; otherwise exact spatial alignment must be achieved (see below). Secondly, because the two images result from the injection of different amounts of activity and are recorded at different times after administration, they have to be normalised in some way before being subtracted. As a result the final image is obtained by the subtraction of a transformed image

$$\text{matrix A} - \text{k (matrix B)} = \text{matrix C}$$

where k is the normalisation factor. Due to statistical variations in count rates after subtraction, some pixels in the image will appear with negative values. These are generally displayed with zero, whilst the target concentration remains highly positive (Figure 5.1b).

One point which should be considered with the use of image subtraction is that the process is removing counts from an image which invariably has unfavourable counting statistics and a high degree of noise at the onset. This should be taken into account when images are visually assessed, particularly regarding the degree of image smoothing and any subsequent processing of the recorded data.

Simulation of Non-Target Activity

As described previously, background subtraction is a correction technique which is intended to increase the contrast of immunoscintigraphic images. A range of radiopharmaceuticals has been employed for this purpose (see Table 5.3). In some cases the background agent is used for subtraction of the whole background area, whilst in others subtraction has been limited to a specific organ of interest such as the liver. Some workers have simply used a second radiopharmaceutical such as Tc-99m-DTPA or Tc-99m-diphosphonate to outline normal structures such as the urinary tract or the skeleton. In these situations the images are simply compared visually to assess sites of abnormal antibody uptake.

If it is performed correctly, background subtraction may be used to increase the confidence of lesion detection. However, if it is incorrectly applied, it may produce misleading information, reducing the diagnostic accuracy of the technique.

A fundamental requirement of this technique is that the distribution of the second radiopharmaceutical should match exactly the non-target distribution of the radiolabelled antibody, although for both biological and physical reasons this is virtually impossible to achieve. For simultaneous imaging by the gamma camera, the principal energies of the gamma rays emitted by the two radiopharmaceuticals must be sufficiently different to be resolved by the pulse height analyser without overlap of the windows. In addition, the contribution from the scatter down from the high-energy photons into the lower-energy window must be negligible. This is normally achieved by the administration of a higher amount of activity of the lower-energy radiopharmaceutical, rendering the amount of any scatter from the high-energy radiopharmaceutical in the lower-energy window insignificant. DeLand et al. (1980) originally stated that the principal gamma energy of the background radiopharma-

TABLE 5.3. Radiopharmaceuticals Suitable for Background Subtraction

Form	Biodistribution	Radionuclide
Irrelevant immunoglobulin	Intravascular and extravascular blood pool	Tc-99m In-111 Ga-67 I-123
Human serum albumin	Intravascular blood pool	Tc-99m
Red blood cells	Intravascular blood pool	Tc-99m
Transferrin	Intravascular blood pool	In-113m
Pertechnetate	Extravascular blood pool Thyroid Stomach Urinary Trace	Tc-99m
Colloid or phytate	Liver	Tc-99m In-111 In-113m
Diphosphonate	Bone	Tc-99m

ceutical should be lower than that of the antibody radiolabel. However, a number of authors have subsequently reported that the subtraction of images of radionuclides having different photon energies results in the production of image artefacts (Ott et al., 1983; Green et al., 1984; Perkins, 1984; Liehn, 1988). A particular problem with this technique has been the generation of subtraction artefacts, particularly at positions which could not be associated with tumours—for example, increased counts resulting at the edges of images and outside the perimeter of the patient. In some cases these artefacts have rendered the images of no clinical value (Ott et al., 1983). However, in that particular study no attempts were made to minimise errors or optimise the imaging conditions. Green et al. (1984) reported that the artefactual positive regions which occurred could be avoided by the experienced observer.

These foci of increased uptake are commonly seen in the area of the stomach, the lower left border of the heart, the lower right border of the left lung, the inferior border of the right lobe of the liver, around any site of recent surgery or trauma, and in the region of the urinary bladder. By working to a set of empirical rules, these artefacts could be recognised and accounted for. Green et al. also went on to prove statistically that background images using Tc-99m-labelled albumin and free pertechnetate were good models for the non-tumour regions and that by comparing the ratios of count rates between the tumour and non-tumour regions in the paired images these regions were shown to form statistically distinct groups.

Assuming a perfect simulation of the biodistribution of the background tracer, image artefacts mainly result from different photon attenuation, collimator septal

penetration, and scatter of the two radionuclides used for radiolabelling the antibody
and background agent. Perkins et al.
(1984) modified the subtraction method in
order to reduce the differential septal penetration and scatter components in the
images. This involved thresholding the antibody image by subtracting a constant
count rate measured in a region of interest
defined outside the border of the patient.
An example of the threshold subtraction
process using I-131-OC125 F(ab')$_2$ fragments and Tc-99m-HSA and free pertechnetate in a patient with a recurrent ovarian
carcinoma is given in Figure 5.2. Other attempts to minimise these energy differences were in the use of a background
agent with a gamma energy more closely
matched to that of the antibody radiolabel,
but this often restricted imaging to a single
view (Perkins et al., 1984; Liehn et al.,
1988). In some cases an early image of the
blood pool distribution of the injected antibody has been used for subtraction
(Granowska et al., 1988). This approach
satisfies the problems of energy differences but introduces a potential source of
error in patient positioning.

Geometric Image Registration

The optimum subtraction of one image
from another is only possible if the image
sizes and spatial alignment are identical.
When viewing images of radionuclides of
different photon energies, it is apparent
that the spatial size of the image varies
with energy. The subtraction of an early
blood pool phase image from a later uptake
image overcomes the problem of energy
differences but does necessitate accurate
repositioning of the views. This is first
carried out by the use of superficial
markers placed on the surface of the patient. Bony landmarks such as xiphister-

num, costal margins, anterior superior
iliac spines, and symphysis pubis are
marked with indelible ink, and a point
source of radioactivity positioned over
these prior to imaging. In this way the
images may be realigned at each visit. Anatomical features such as large vessels may
also be used to aid realignment. Fine registration of the images is then carried out by
computer following acquisition of the data.
The images may be moved a pixel at a time
vertically, horizontally, or by rotation. The
images may then be subtracted following
normalisation of the count rates. These
images may also be analysed by computer
for the assessment of any dynamic change
in biodistribution (kinetic analysis). The
main criticism of this procedure using
image realignment is that although the surface markers on any one patient are relatively fixed, the positions of internal organs and structures will vary greatly with
time. For example, the positions of abdominal organs will vary with distension of the
stomach following meals and the degree of
fullness of the urinary bladder. In the case
of colon cancer in particular, barium X-ray
and radionuclide whole bowel transit studies have shown the large range of move-
ments of the bowel. Hence the subtraction
of images recorded at different times
should be restricted to the diagnosis of lesions that are known to be fixed in relation
to the surface markers used.

Image Normalisation

The biodistribution of the tracers used
for paired image subtraction may differ
greatly because of defects or active zones,
resulting, for example, from differences in
vascular permeability of the tracers. The
effect of normalisation on the subtracted
images is therefore complicated. The normalisation step is necessary to adjust the

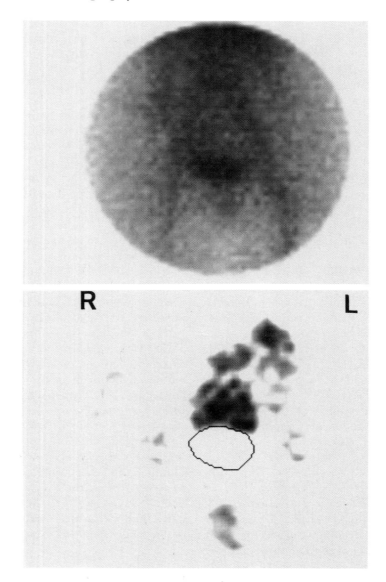

Fig. 5.2. Anterior images of the lower abdomen and pelvis of a patient with a large recurrent carcinoma of the ovary recorded 48 h following administration of 80 MBq I-131-OC125F(ab')$_2$. **Top:** Antibody image 200 K counts. A 600 K count image was recorded simultaneously following administration of 200 MBq Tc-99m-HSA and 200 MBq Tc-99mO$_4^-$. **Bottom:** Threshold subtraction image showing region of tumour uptake. A region of interest is drawn on the images to show the position of the bladder.

images for the difference in the total number of recorded counts due to the variable acquisition parameters of the study. The normalisation factor may be obtained in a variety of ways from the recorded images. In general this may be obtained by obtaining the ratio of the total number of counts in the two images or by selecting an appropriate region of interest, such as the heart or liver. Jackson et al. (1985) used the ratio of radioactivity in two blood samples taken at the time of imaging to calculate the normalisation factor.

The numerical value obtained will dramatically affect the appearance of the final subtracted image, and unless some form of automatic normalisation routine is used, the results will be variable. The use of an iterative automatic normalisation method has a great deal of merit. Venot et al. (1983) adopted an iterative automated method of image normalisation first used in nuclear medicine for pancreas imaging (Skretting, 1975). This was based on a unidimensional optimisation method known as the Fibonacci search. This routine permits a number of subtracted images within a range of normalisation factors, typically 0 and 200%. As described earlier, following image subtraction because of the presence of noise in the images, the pixel values in the non-target areas of the subtraction image do not equal zero but exhibit random fluctuations, either positive or negative. This processing routine counts the sign changes in each pixel of the subtracted image, line by line. For example,

$$++ - +++ -- +   R = 4$$

and

$$-- ++ - + -- +++ -   R = 6.$$

The normalisation factor is automatically taken from the subtracted image with the greatest R value. This approach has been evaluated in detail by Liehn et al. (1987, 1988).

Kinetic Analysis and Probability Mapping

By examining the dynamic information in paired or sequential images, it is feasible to map out the spatial distribution of temporal variations in image activity. This is based on the different kinetics of tumour uptake and blood and normal tissue clearance which occurs over a period of time following the initial distribution phase. Similar algorithms have been adopted for the detection of temporal changes in the spatial uniformity of the gamma camera detector response. Granowska et al. (1988) have reported the use of this technique comparing images recorded at 10 minutes or 4 hours with images recorded at 22 hours using I-123 antibody for the detection of ovarian carcinoma, where biopsy proven deposits of 0.5 cm diameter have been identified. This technique does have the potential for being particularly sensitive; however, it is subject to errors in patient realignment and superposition of paired images, especially with regard to the movement of internal body structures as described previously. In cases of tumour recurrence where tissues are fixed due to adhesions, this technique could be of most benefit.

SECOND ANTIBODY CLEARANCE

The main source of background radioactivity in the patient is in the form of radiolabelled antibody in the circulation. An alternative to the use of computer-assisted image subtraction to reduce background activity is the use of a second antibody directed against the first tumour associated antibody to promote clearance from the circulation. This was first described by Begent et al. (1982), using a liposomally entrapped second antibody which resulted in a two-to-four-fold acceleration of the clearance of the radiolabelled antibody from the circulation. The clearance in these studies was mainly to the liver, a feature which has since been attributed to the use of liposomes which are known to accumulate in the reticuloendothelial system. The use of liposomes is not essential however. Other work using anti-CEA antibody in hamsters (Sharkey et al., 1984) and in patients (Goodwin et al., 1984) have also shown the use of a second antibody to result in accelerated whole body clearance of radiolabelled antibody without such an intense accumulation in the liver. In most cases the second antibody is an anti-species antibody, i.e., if murine antibody is used, a goat anti-mouse antibody could be used. Sharkey et al. (1984) used a radiolabelled goat polyclonal anti-CEA antibody with a donkey anti-goat IgG second antibody for their experiments.

Given that satisfactory imaging is possible using some radiolabelled antibodies alone, it seems unlikely that this technique will be widely used. Problems of patient sensitisation to foreign immunoglobulins are likely to restrict the administration of second antibody for diagnostic imaging.

ANTIBODY EMISSION TOMOGRAPHY

Planar imaging techniques are restricted to the visualisation of distributions in three-dimensional space using two-dimensional projections. Although some depth information may be obtained from planar views and lateral and oblique views may also be acquired, data recorded by single photon emission computed tomography (SPECT) have significant theoretical advantages over data recorded in a single plane. This has been shown in some nuclear medicine investigations—for example, tomography of brain, myocardium, liver, and bone—although in some cases SPECT has been only of limited value. The main theoretical advantages of SPECT are improved image contrast, information with depth, and the quantification of data in the individual slice or tomogram being studied (Jarritt and Ell, 1984). Experimental studies using phantoms have demonstrated a significant increase in lesion-to-background contrast using SPECT (Jaszczak et al., 1982), and this has an important bearing on the clinical use of radiolabelled antibodies. The gain in contrast resolution over planar scintigraphy is an important factor because of the relatively low T:NT uptake of antibodies currently in use. Visualisation of the antibody distribution slice by slice allows recognition of other sites of non-specific uptake such as liver, spleen, kidneys, and bladder, thus increasing sensitivity.

Detailed published studies on the use of antibody emission tomography are limited. From the few clinical studies that have been reported, an increase in sensitivity using SPECT has been apparent, although many variable factors affect the performance of the technique (Mach et al., 1981; Berche et al., 1982; Bares et al., 1987; Perkins et al., 1988). Studies carried out by Bares et al. (1987) compared SPECT with planar imaging using I-131- and In-111-labelled anti-CEA antibodies and showed an increase in the sensitivity of tumour detection from 50% to 87%. Studies by Epenetos et al. (1982) using I-123-labelled antibodies against milk fat globule membrane (HMFG1 and HMFG2) described the use of emission tomography to aid in the identification of antibody uptake in pelvic tumours in close proximity to radioiodide in the urinary bladder. Perkins et al. (1988) carried out a detailed comparison of planar and SPECT tumour imaging using I-131 and In-111-labelled antibody. In general, the authors found unsatisfactory results using I-131 antibodies, mainly due to low count rates and the necessity for long acquisition times of up to 1 hour, which are not possible in busy departments. The use of SPECT for monitoring the biodistribution of therapeutic doses of I-131-labelled antibodies would not be subject to these restrictions since the administered doses would be greater. However, it is recommended that specially designed collimators are used for this purpose (Clarke et al., 1985).

In general, the use of SPECT imaging using In-111 and Tc-99m as the radiolabel has been found to increase tumour detection from sensitivities of the order of 70% to about 90%. The authors have previously reported a two-fold increase in T:NT image contrast measured from planar and SPECT images of the thorax of patients administered with In-111-labelled antibody (Perkins et al., 1988).

SPECT Data Collection and Reconstruction

The majority of nuclear medicine departments use rotating gamma cameras for tomographic imaging. Equipment used for these studies must perform to high technical standards and be regularly calibrated using appropriate phantoms. Most gamma cameras are designed primarily for the use of Tc-99m, and it is therefore to be expected that the best results would be obtained using either this radionuclide or I-123, which has a similar energy. The choice of collimator is obviously important in this respect, and it is important that the camera gantry is stable during rotation if heavy collimators are used for higher energy radionuclides. The following parameters are particularly important with

respect to gamma camera emission tomography:

1. Inhomogeneity of detector response
2. Alignment of the centre of rotation
3. Gamma ray attenuation

In most instances individual centres will need to perform calibration studies on their own equipment to determine the optimum parameters for data collection and reconstruction. It is preferable if uniformity correction is carried out using a source of the same radionuclide that is used for the antibody radiolabel. Correction with an appropriate gamma ray attenuation factor will be necessary with lower energy radionuclides such as Tc-99m and I-123, but this will not be so important in the case of I-131 or In-111. Typical parameters for imaging are shown in Table 5.4. These values give an approximate guide to the imaging times and the count rates which may be obtained and should only be used as a guideline as they ultimately depend upon the type and performance of equipment. The total numbers of recorded counts will depend upon the region of the body being imaged, and the number of counts in each view will depend on the number of slices reconstructed, commonly 32 or 64, representing a slice thickness of 12.5 or 6.3 mm, respectively.

Data is typically recorded throughout a full 360-degree rotation using 64 incremental steps and may be reconstructed to view axial, coronal, and sagittal slices, all of which can add useful information to the study. In general, reconstruction of data should be performed using a filter with a high degree of smoothing such as a Hann filter. In the authors' experience it is often necessary to carry out further smoothing of the images in three dimensions.

TABLE 5.4. Typical Parameters for SPECT Imaging

Radiolabel	Administered dose (MBq)	Time of imaging	Data collection time	Total counts collected
I-131	80–120	48–72 h	<60 min	<5 M
In-111	80–120	48–72 h	20–40 min	5 M
I-123	30–300	<24 h	20–40 min	5 M
Tc-99m	1000	<24 h	20–30 min	5–10 M

Smoothing in this way is generally preferable to the addition of slices to obtain cuts with higher counts.

Clinical Utility of SPECT Imaging

There is mixed opinion regarding the clinical utility of SPECT for routine antibody imaging. The advances that have recently been reported in the use of In-111-, I-123-, and Tc-99m-labelled antibodies have resulted in dramatic improvements in the quality of planar images. In the majority of instances, SPECT imaging is valuable in confirming uptake in lesions suspected on planar views or in identifying sites of false positive uptake such as excretion into the bowel or urinary bladder. Reports of use of In-111 have probably been the most favourable (Perkins et al., 1988, Britton et al., 1988), although high liver uptake restricts the use of this radiolabel mainly to imaging sites within the thorax, lower abdomen, and pelvis. One of the smallest lesions visualised in studies performed by the authors was in a patient with lung metastases from osteogenic sarcoma. Planar imaging of the chest failed to demonstrate an abnormality, whereas a 10 mm metastasis in the left lung was visualised in an axial view through the thorax (Fig. 5.3). Liver uptake is clearly a disadvantage of In-111 and Tc-99m-labelled antibody; however, tracer uptake in the bone marrow provides valuable anatomical reference markers for localisation of lesions.

Despite problems of low count rates for imaging, it is essential that tomography is achieved in relatively short acquisition periods. In most cases patients undergoing imaging studies are unfit and are often unable to lie still for long periods. It is therefore desirable that imaging should be performed in the minimum of time, and a period of 20–30 minutes is generally considered acceptable for most patients. Increasing data acquisition time will only increase the likelihood of patient movement, thus negating the value of the study. The ultimate resolution of the imaging technique will only improve with the development of antibodies or fragments with increased specificity. In the majority of imaging studies, antibody imaging is still not capable of demonstrating tumours smaller that 5–10 mm diameter. This represents large populations of the order of 10^{13} tumour cells (Lentle et al., 1985). Clearly this represents an advanced stage of disease. There is great room for improvement both in terms of radiopharmaceutical design and equipment performance. No doubt these advances will be paralleled with advances in X-ray CT and magnetic resonance imaging. The presentation of SPECT antibody images in the same orien-

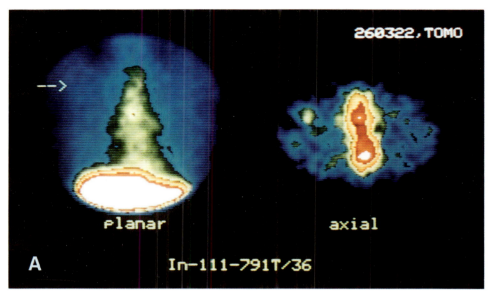

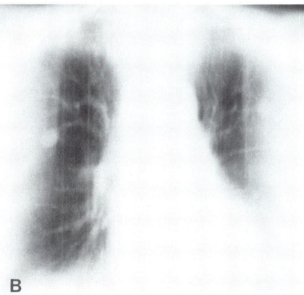

Fig. 5.3. A: Anterior planar (left) and axial view (right) of the thorax of patient with lung metastases from osteogenic sarcoma recorded 72 h following administration of 80 MBq In-111-791T/36 antibody. Intense liver uptake was seen in the planar view but, despite windowing the display no abnormality was visible. The axial cut at the position of the horizontal line shows activity posteriorly within the thoracic vertebrae and uptake in a 10 mm diameter metastasis in the mid zone of the right lung. B: No abnormality was visible in a plain chest radiograph. However, following the antibody study a tomographic radiograph demonstrated two metastases in the lungs. The metastasis in the left lung was not visualised in the antibody study.

tations as images from these other imaging modalities will establish the complementary nature of these investigations.

REFERENCES AND FURTHER READING

Bares, R., Fass, J., Buell, V., Schumpelick, V. (1987): Validity of tomographical methods for radioimmunodetection of gastrointestinal tumours. In: Klapdor, R. (ed.): "New Tumour Markers and Their Monoclonal Antibodies." Stuttgart: Georg Thieme, pp. 470–474.

Begent, R.H., Green, A.J., Bagshawe, K.D., Jones, B.E., Keep, P.A., Searle, F., Jewkes, R.F., Barratt, G.M., Ryman, B.E. (1982): Liposomally entrapped second antibody improves tumour imaging with radiolabelled (first) antitumour antibody. Lancet II: 739–742.

Beihn, R.M., Damron, J.R., Hafner, T. (1974): Subtraction technique for the detection of subphrenic abscesses using 67 Ga and Tc-99m. J. Nucl. Med. 15:371–373.

Berche, C., Mach, J-P., Lumbroso, J-D., Langlais, C., Aubry, F., Buchegger, F., Carrel, S., Rougier, P., Parmentier, C., Tubiana, M. (1982): Tomoscintigraphy for detecting gastrointestinal and medullary thyroid cancers: First clinical results using radiolabelled monoclonal antibodies against carcinoembryonic antigen. B.M.J. 285:1447–1451.

Bradwell, A.R., Taylor, J.R., Fairweather, D.S., Chandler, S., Dykes, P.W. (1983): Model for the radioimmunodetection of tumours. Protides of the Biological Fluids 31:313–316.

Bradwell, A.R., Fairweather, D.S., Dykes, P.W. (1985): Developments in antibody imaging. In: Baldwin, R.W., Byers, V.S. (eds.): Monoclonal Antibodies for Cancer Detection and Therapy. New York: Academic Press, pp. 65–85.

Britton, K.E., Buragg, G.L., Bares, R., Bischof-Delaloye, A., Buell, U., Emrich, D., Granowska, M. (1989): A brief guide to the practice of radioimmunoscintigraphy and radioimmunotherapy in cancer. Int. J. Biol. Markers 4:106–118.

Clarke, L.P., Saw, C.B., Leong, L.K., Serafini, N.K. (1985): SPECT imaging of ^{131}I (364keV): Importance of collimation. Nucl. Med. Commun. 6:41–47.

Deland, F.H., Kim, E.E., Simmons, G., Goldenberg, D.M. (1980): Imaging approach in radioimmunodetection. Cancer Res. 40:3046–3049.

Epenetos, A.A., Britton, K.E., Mather, S., Shepherd, J., Granowska, M., Taylor-Papadimitriou, J., Nimmon, C.C., Durbin, H., Hawkins, L.R., Malpas, J.S., Bodmer, W.F. (1982): Targeting of iodine-123-labelled tumour-associated monoclonal antibodies to ovarian, breast and gastrointestinal tumours. Lancet II:999–1004.

Fairweather, D.S., Irwin, M., Bradwell, A.R., Dykes, P.W., Flinn, R.H. (1983): Computer analysis of antibody scans. Protides of Biological Fluids 31:285–288.

Farrands, P.A., Perkins, A.C., Pimm, M.V., Hardy, J.D., Embleton, M.J., Baldwin, R.W., Hardcastle, J.D. (1982): Radioimmunodetection of human colorectal cancers by an anti-tumour monoclonal antibody. Lancet II:397–400.

Ferlin, G., Borsato, N., Camerani, M., Conte, N., Zotti, D. (1983): New perspectives in localizing enlarged parathyroids by technetium-thallium subtraction scan. J. Nucl. Med. 24:438–441.

Goldenberg, D.M., DeLand, F.H. (1982): History and status of tumour imaging with radiolabelled antibodies. J. Biol. Response Mod. 1:121–136.

Goldenberg, D.M., Deland, F., Kim, E., Bennett, S., Primus, F.J., van Nagell, J.E., Estes, N., DeSimone, P., Rayburn, P. (1978): Use of radiolabeled antibodies to carcinoembryonig antigen for the detection and localization of diverse cancers by external photoscanning. New. Engl. J. Med. 298:1384–1388.

Goldenberg, D.M., Kim, E.E., Deland, F.H., Bennett, S., Primus, F.J. (1980): Radioimmunodetection of cancer with radioactive antibodies to carcinoembryonic antigen. Cancer Res. 40:2984–2992.

Goodwin, D., Meares, C., Diamanti, C., McCall, M., Lai, C., Torti, F., McTigue, M., Martin, B. (1984): Use of specific antibody for rapid clearance of circulating blood background from radiolabeled tumor imaging proteins. Eur. J. Nucl. Med. 9:209–215.

Goris, M.L., Briandet, P.A. (1983): A clinical and mathematical introduction to computer processing of scintigraphic images. New York: Raven Press.

Granowska, M., Nimmon, C.C., Britton, K.E. (1988): Kinetic analysis and probability mapping applied to the detection of ovarian cancer by radioimmunoscintigraphy. J. Nucl. Med. 29:599–607.

Granowska, M., Nimmon, C.C., Britton, K.E., Crowther, M., Mather, S.J., Slevin, M.L., Shepherd, J.H. (1988): Kinetic analysis and probability mapping applied to the detection of ovarian cancer by radioimmunoscintigraphy. J. Nucl. Med. 29: 599–607.

Green, A.J., Begent, R.H., Keep, P.A., Bagshawe, K.D. (1984): Analysis of radioimmunodetection of tumors by the subtraction technique. J. Nucl. Med. 25:96–100.

Jackson, P.C., Pitcher, E.M., Davies, J.O., Davies, E.R., Sadowski, C.S., Staddon, G.E., Stirrat, G.M., Sunderland, C.A. (1985): Radionuclide imaging of ovarian tumours with a radiolabelled (I-123) monoclonal antibody (NDOG2). Eur. J. Nucl. Med. 11:22–28.

Jarritt, P.H., Ell, P.J. (1984): Gamma camera emission computed tomography. Quality control and clinical applications. London: Current Medical Literature Ltd.

Jaszczak, R.J., Whitehead, F.R., Kim, C.B., Coleman, R.E. (1982): Lesion detection with single photon emission computed tomography (SPECT) compared with conventional imaging. J. Nucl. Med. 26:531–537.

Kaplan, E., Ben-Porath, M., Fink, S., Clayton, G.D., Jacobson, B. (1966): Elimination of liver interference from the selenomethionine pancreas. Scan. J. Nucl. Med. 7:807–816.

Lakshmanan, A.V., Sharp, P., Mallard, J. (1978): The influence of size and radiopharmaceutical concentration ratio on the detection of abnormalities in clinical radionuclide imaging. Br. J. Radiol. 51:986–991.

Larsson, S.A. (1980): Gamma camera emission tomography. Acta Radiologica Supplementum 363.

Lentle, B.C., Scott, J.R., Schmidt, R.P., Hooper, H.R., Catz, Z. (1985): The clinical value of direct tumour scintigraphy: A new hypothesis. J. Nucl. Med. 26:1215–1217.

Liehn, J.C. (1988): Image subtraction techniques in immunoscintigraphy. In: Srivastara, S.C. (ed.): "Radiolabelled Monoclonal Antibodies for Imaging and Therapy." New York: Plenum Publishing Co., pp. 513–540.

Liehn, J.C., Hannequin, P., Nasea, S., Lebrun, D., Cattan, A., Valeyre, J. (1987): A new approach to image subtraction in immunoscintigraphy: Preliminary results. Eur. J. Nucl. Med. 13:391–396.

Mach, J.P., Buchegger, F., Forni, M., Ritschard, J., Berche, C., Lumbroso, J.D., Schreyer, J., Girardet, C., Accolla, R.S., Carrel, S. (1981): Use of radiolabelled monoclonal anti-CEA antibodies for the detection of human carcinomas by external photoscanning and tomoscintigraphy. Immunol. Today 239–249.

Ott, R.J., Grey, L.J., Zivanovic, M.A., Flower, M.A., Trott, N.G., Moshakis, V., Coombes, R.C., Neville, A.M., Ormerod, M.G., Westwood, J.H., McCready, V.R. (1983): The limitation of the dual radionuclide subtraction technique for the external detection of tumours by radioiodine-labelled antibodies. Br. J. Radiol. 56:101–108.

Perkins, A.C., Whalley, D.R., Ballantyne, K.C., Pimm, M.V. (1988): Gamma camera emission tomography using radiolabelled antibodies. Eur. J. Nucl. Med. 14:45–49.

Perkins, A.C., Whalley, D.R., Hardy, J.G. (1984): Physical approach for the reduction of dual radionuclide image subtraction artifacts in immunoscintigraphy. Nucl. Med. Commun. 5:501–512.

Rockoff, S.D., Goodenough, D.J., McIntire, K.R. (1980): Theoretical limitations in the immunodiagnostic imaging of cancer with computed tomography and nuclear scanning. Cancer Res. 40:3054–3058.

Rollo, F.D., Patton, J.A. (1980): Imaging techniques for the radioimmunodetection of cancer. Cancer Res. 40:3050–3053.

Sharkey, R.M., Primus, F.J., Goldenberg, D.M. (1984): Second antibody clearance of radiolabeled antibody in cancer radioimmunodetection. Proc. Natl. Acad. Sci. USA. 81:2843–2846.

Skretting, A., Aas, M., Normann, E., Sodal, G., Lindegaard, M.W. (1978): Clinical results with ^{131}I-toluidine blue and triple radionuclide subtraction for preoperative localization of enlarged parathyroid glands. Eur. J. Nucl. Med. 3:5–9.

Venot, A., Lebrucheck, J.F., Golmard, J.L., Roucayrol, J.C. (1983): An automated method for the normalization of scintigraphic images. J. Nucl. Med. 24:412–422.

Venot, A., Golmard, J.L., Lebruchec, J.F., Pronzato, L., Walter, E., Fril, G., Roucayrol, J.C. (1984): Digital methods for change detection in medical images. In: Deconinck, F. (ed.): Information Processing in Medical Imaging." The Hague: Martinus Nijhoff, pp. 1–16.

Wahl, R.L., Tuscan, M.C., Botti, J.M. (1986): Dynamic variable background subtraction: A simple means of displaying radiolabeled monoclonal antibody scintigrams. J. Nucl. Med. 27:545–548.

6 Immunological Responses to Monoclonal Antibodies

INTRODUCTION

When murine monoclonal antibodies are injected into patients, they are recognised by the body as foreign proteins and are capable of initiating an immune response. The antibody being administered may be capable of behaving as an antigen against which anti-antibodies may be produced. These anti-antibodies can be found circulating in the patient's blood stream and can be detected in plasma or serum using an appropriate assay. It is known that some healthy individuals possess antibodies directed against various animal proteins, and in some cases pre-existing anti-mouse antibodies capable of reacting with murine immunoglobulin have been detected in blood samples taken from patients. However, in these instances the pre-existing anti-mouse antibodies are directed towards the Fc portion of the antibody molecule. These are probably cross-reacting antibodies initially generated in response to exposure to animals or animal immunoglobulins in the diet. Rheumatoid factor, an anti-immunoglobulin antibody directed against denatured IgG and present in the serum of some individuals with rheumatoid arthritis, may also cross react with foreign immunoglobulins such as monoclonal antibodies. The effects of these type of antibodies on monoclonal antibodies administered to patients for immunoscintigraphy is at the present time largely unknown.

The true human anti-mouse antibody generated in response to exposure to murine antibody is known as human anti-mouse antibody (HAMA). The resulting immune response may be of practical significance for the patient, especially if the response is severe and the patient becomes hypersensitive. In the majority of clinical studies to date murine monoclonal antibody preparations have been used, thus stimulating an HAMA response. However, the more recent introduction of humanised monoclonal antibodies has raised the theoretical possibility of the production of human anti-human antibody (HAHA).

During the 1980s the use of radiolabelled antibodies for imaging both malignant and benign conditions increased dramatically. The number of commercially

111

available preparations is growing steadily, with most radiopharmaceutical companies offering at least one monoclonal antibody-based radiopharmaceutical for *in vivo* use. The growing trend for using monoclonal antibodies for non-malignant conditions, such as in myocardial infarction, using anti-myosin antibody and in cell labelling (e.g., P256 platelet-specific antibody and BW250/183 anti-granulocyte antibody) has exposed a new and expanding population of patients to murine immunoglobulin. In subsequent years this patient population may face immunological problems as a result of further antibody-based investigations or immunotherapy for other, life threatening, diseases.

ANTIBODY RESPONSE

The primary antibody response following the first injection of an antigen such as a monoclonal antibody may be divided into four phases: A lag phase usually of about 2 days, but which may last as long as 10 or 12 days during which no response is observed; a log phase usually of about 2 weeks duration when the induced anti-antibody titres rise logarithmically; a plateau phase, where titres level out; and finally, a decline phase when the anti-antibodies are catabolized or cleared as complexes of antibody and anti-antibody. The time course of the immune response events varies from patient to patient and cannot be predicted. HAMA has been detected in blood samples taken from patients as early as 7 days following administration of monoclonal antibody for diagnostic imaging, and this has been observed to persist in the circulation for over two years. The major component of the initial primary response is the production of IgM antibodies followed by IgG production.

If a patient receives a repeat injection of monoclonal antibody, this causes most of their antibody-producing B lymphocytes to switch from IgM production to IgG production, which then gives rise to very high IgG titres in the circulation. In addition, it has been observed that the affinity of antibodies increases during the secondary response (affinity maturation). In some cases the process of sensitisation which takes place in the patient is also accompanied by the production of IgE, which becomes fixed to Fc receptors on mast cells. However this is variable, depending upon the state of the individual and the characteristics of the antibody preparation administered.

INTERACTIONS OF HAMA WITH MONOCLONAL ANTIBODIES

The exact nature of the induced antibody response to monoclonal antibodies is complicated and poorly understood. A wide range of variable factors, such as the antibody isotype, fragments, administered protein dose, and the condition of the patients, including their individual immunocompetence and any pre-existing levels of anti-antibody in the circulation, need to be considered. Correlation of these factors is fraught with problems, and the reader is recommended to refer to a literature review published by Van Kroonenbergh and Pauwels (1988).

The HAMA response may be directed against both the variable and constant regions of the antibody molecule. This may consist of IgM, IgG, anti-isotypic, anti-idiotypic, and anti-species antibodies, all of which have been detected in the sera of patients administered with monoclonal antibodies for diagnostic imaging. Once HAMA has been induced, it is capable of neutralising the effects of subsequent doses of administered antibody by reducing bioavailability due to the formation of immune complexes of monoclonal antibody and HAMA.

These immune complexes are cleared by the cells of the reticuloendothelial system, particularly the liver and spleen. It is therefore the second and subsequent administration of monoclonal antibody which may present the greatest problems for the diagnostic and therapeutic use of monoclonal antibodies. The repeated use of antibodies for diagnostic imaging will increase the possibility of HAMA production. The possible effects of such procedures are mainly an alteration of image quality and the possibility of hypersensitive reactions, as described subsequently. In addition it should also be appreciated that the presence of HAMA in the circulation may interfere with *in vitro* immunoassays that use an antibody of murine origin, and false results may be obtained.

IMAGING CONSEQUENCES OF HAMA
Clinical Studies

In medical oncology the evolving role for immunoscintigraphy would appear to be the detection of secondary and recurrent disease. Such diagnostic strategies inevitably involve repeat imaging investigations during patient follow-up, and therefore the possibility of patient sensitisation against the administered immunoradiopharmaceuticals will be increased. Even with the low amounts of protein (<10 mg) usually administered for diagnostic imaging, an HAMA response may be detected following the first administered dose of antibody. This has also been observed in the case of $F(ab')_2$ and Fab fragments. Such responses may lead to problems when subsequent doses are administered. The production of HAMA may result in changes in the pharmacokinetic behaviour of the administered antibody. For example, it is considered that HAMA may stimulate the

removal of antibody by the reticuloendothelial system in the form of complexes. Clinical studies have shown that patients with detectable HAMA levels in the circulation will clear radiolabelled antibody from the bloodstream more rapidly than those with no detectable HAMA. From work carried out by the authors, it is evident that the distribution of radiolabel visualised by the gamma camera in the presence of a HAMA response is different for indium and iodine labelled antibody. Repeat studies using I-131-labelled antibody have shown increased concentration of radiolabel in the spleen (see Fig. 6.1), whereas with In-111-labelled antibody a dramatic increase in liver activity has been observed. In the latter case, this uptake may be visualised as early as 20 minutes following intravenous injection (see Fig. 6.2).

It is not clear whether this difference is due to the different physiological fates of the radionuclides following complex breakdown and clearance or whether different antibody responses are evoked to antibody conjugates with radioiodine or radiometal chelates. Certainly it has been demonstrated in animal studies that radiometal chelate complexes such as DTPA anhydride are themselves immunogenic. It is therefore possible that patients may recognise immunogenically this part of antibodies radiolabelled with metallic radionuclides.

The use of radiopharmaceutical preparations based on antibody fragments has been advocated by some workers as a means of reducing the problems of HAMA production. However, the use of antibody fragments has not always had the desired effect. For example, $F(ab')_2$ fragments of the antibody OC125 are known to highly be immunogenic. Such is the nature of the patient response following intravenous administration of this particular antibody

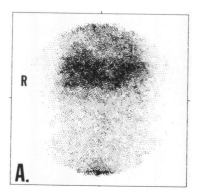

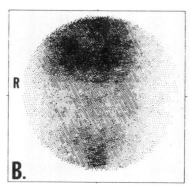

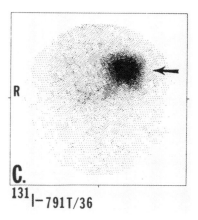

^{131}I–791T/36

Fig. 6.1. Anterior images of the upper abdomen of a 68-year-old patient with a carcinoma of the endometrium. A: 48 hours following the first injection of I-131-791T/36 antibody. B: 3 weeks later and 48 hours following the second injection of I-131-791T/36 antibody. C: 6 months following the first injection of and 48 hours following the third injection of I-131-791T/36 antibody, showing intense uptake in the spleen. In each case the dose of antibody was 200 μg and a subcutaneous skin test was performed prior

that its use in the detection of the benign condition of endometriosis has been contraindicated. Figure 6.3 shows the change in biodistribution between the first, second, and third imaging investigations using F(ab')$_2$ fragments of OC125 antibody labelled with In-111. The patient showed no signs of hypersensitivity on the occasion of the second or third antibody study.

Further clinical information is required before the nature and magnitude of immune responses to monoclonal antibodies are fully realised. In some cases there have been very few reports of HAMA production following administration of monoclonal antibodies. In particular, the use of anti-myosin antibody fragments and antibody fragments for cell labelling studies have resulted in very few instances of detectable HAMA production. One reason for this may be the nature of antibody clearance in the case of antibodies specific for cells or substances encountered in the circulation. In such instances the antibody may not be in a form capable of producing an immune response for a long enough period before reaching its target antigen.

In some cases where an immune response is present the change in biodistribution on repeat administration of a radiolabelled monoclonal antibody may be unexpected and dramatic. Figure 6.4 shows intense hepatic uptake in a patient with colorectal cancer who was injected with 1 mg of intact In-111-labelled anti-CEA (C46, IgG2a) monoclonal antibody three years following administration of In-111-labelled 791T/36 antibody (IgG2b). Even though a subcutaneous skin test was negative prior to the second dose of antibody, the patient collapsed with an immediate (type 1) hypersensitive reaction within 5 minutes of injection of the second dose.

to antibody administration. The site of the tumour was not visualised without blood pool subtraction.

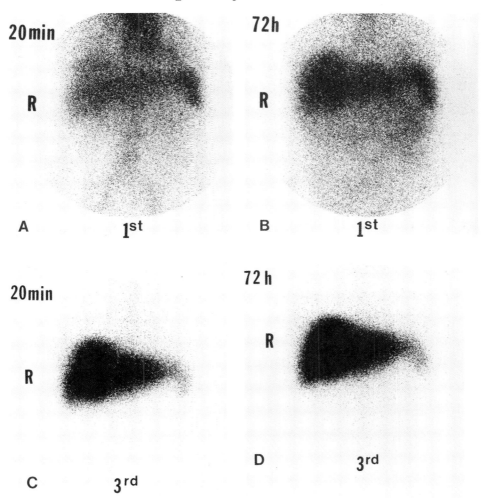

Fig. 6.2. Anterior images of the abdomen of a 69-year-old patient imaged with a suspicion of recurrent ovarian carcinoma. A: 20 minutes and B: 72 hours following the first injection of 1 mg (80 MBq) In-111-791T/36 antibody. C: 20 minutes and D: 72 hours following the third injection of antibody (1 mg (80 MBq) In-111-791T/36) administered 12 months following the first study. A dose of 200 μg I-131-791T/36 antibody was administered 8 months following the first study and no abnormal distribution was observed (images not shown). (From the authors' unpublished studies.)

An important question arising from these observations is whether repeat antibody imaging studies are capable of detecting abnormality with the same accuracy as studies performed following a single administration. Figure 6.5 shows an example of images from a patient with a primary rectal carcinoma which was detected by using In-111-791T/36 antibody.

This patient subsequently developed local recurrence which was successfully detected using In-111-C46 antibody despite the presence of HAMA. Other published data show that true positive imaging results are feasible in the presence of a HAMA response but that the accuracy of lesion detection may be reduced with increased administration of antibody (Per-

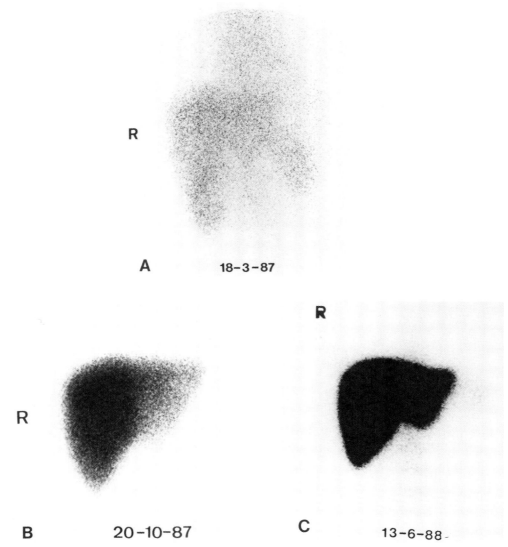

Fig. 6.3. Anterior images of the upper abdomen of a 53-year-old female patient undergoing serial immunoscintigraphy for the investigation of recurrent ovarian carcinoma. Each study was performed 48 hours after the administration of 1 mg (80 MBq) OC125 F(ab')$_2$ antibody. A subcutaneous skin test was performed prior to each intravenous administration. A: initial study showing normal distribution in the liver and kidneys. B: Follow up study 7 months later showing increased hepatic uptake. C: Follow up study 15 months later showing dramatic uptake by the liver. (From the authors' unpublished studies.)

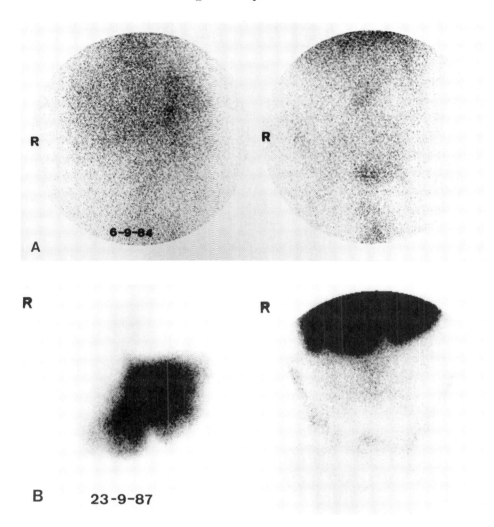

Fig. 6.4. **A**: Anterior images of the upper (**left**) and lower (**right**) abdomen of a 72-year-old male patient with a primary colorectal carcinoma recorded 48 hours following administration of 200 μg (80 MBq) I-131-791T/36 antibody. **B**: Anterior images of the same patient (upper abdomen **right**, lower abdomen **left**) imaged 3 years later for suspected tumour recurrence. The images which show massive hepatic uptake were recorded 48 hours following 1 mg (80 MBq) In-111-C46 anti-CEA antibody. The patient had not received any antibody in the intervening period. (From the authors' unpublished studies.)

kins et al., 1988). However, in some cases it has been claimed that the presence of HAMA may increase the sensitivity of lesion detection. Ford et al. (1988) observed that in some patients with rapidly rising HAMA titres the accelerated clearance of radiolabelled antibody from the circula-

tion reduced the background activity, thus improving tumour visualisation.

Experimental Studies

Since HAMA may impose a serious constraint on the clinical use of murine mono-

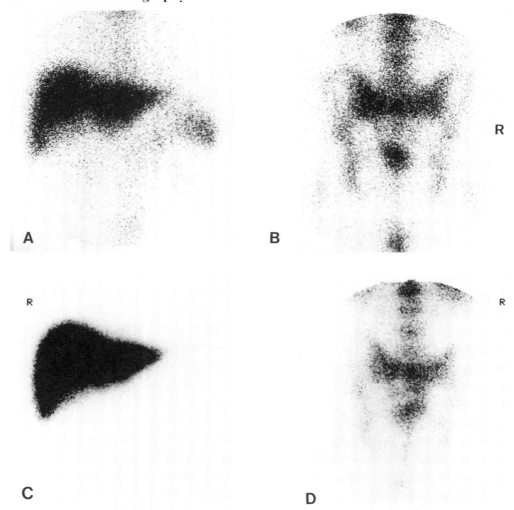

Fig. 6.5. Images of a 43-year-old male patient investigated with a primary tumour of the rectum 48 hours following the administration of 1 mg (80 MBq) In-111-791T/36 antibody. A: anterior view of the liver. B: posterior view of the pelvis showing bone marrow activity and uptake in the tumour low in the pelvis. Images of the same patient two years later, investigated with 1 mg (80 MBq) In-111-C46 antibody. C: anterior view of the liver. D: posterior view of the pelvis. Despite increased hepatic uptake of the tracer the tumour recurrence (which was confirmed at surgery) could be clearly seen. (From the authors' unpublished studies.)

clonal antibodies for diagnosis and therapy, it is important that the characteristics of the antibody response is fully understood. Serological analysis will provide data on the nature of the responses, and in addition the use of an animal model offers a great deal to the understanding of the bio-

logical consequences of HAMA on subsequent antibody administrations. Although marmosets and rabbits have been examined in this context, a rat model has been shown to be of value for imaging studies (Pimm et al., 1988). This model is suitable for the examination of the biological effects of repeat doses of antibody and has provided valuable data on the use of different routes of injection, different antibody isotypes, and the use of immunosuppressive techniques.

In particular, it is important that the animal model used is suitable for imaging studies. In the case of the rat, the major organs may be identified during imaging with a gamma camera fitted with a parallel hole collimator, thus permitting visual examination of any alteration in biodistribution resulting from the presence of anti-mouse antibody (AMA). The use of the gamma camera is of particular value since imaging studies provide relatively large amounts of data from a small group of animals without resorting to killing the animals for dissection. In addition, it is possible to measure the titre of the antibody response in serum from the rats taken at various time points in the study. In this way the AMA titre may be related to the imaging results.

Doses of antibody should be scaled down to an equivalent body weight basis such that a patient dose of a few milligrams would be represented by an experimental dose of the order of 50-100 μg/kg. Specific activities of radiolabelled preparations similar to those in clinical use should also be used. Gamma camera imaging of rats following the first intravenous injection of radiolabelled antibody enables visualisation of the normal distribution of the immunoradiopharmaceutical. In the case of In-111-labelled antibody of the order of 30–40% of the whole body, radioactivity may be found in the liver within 4 to 5 hours following injection. Studies carried out by the authors have shown that a substantial but variable proportion of rats previously sensitised to mouse monoclonal antibody subsequently exhibit a marked perturbation in the biodistribution of subsequent doses of radiolabelled antibody, these finding being consistent with clinical studies.

In rats with a positive response, imaging studies have shown over 90% of the surviving whole body radioactivity to be contained within the liver. Of particular interest were the findings that in cases where rats had been sensitised to one particular antibody (In-111-791T/36), there was a similar perturbation of the In-111-labelled Fab fragment of the same antibody and of another antibody of the same isotype (IgG2b). In contrast there was little influence on the biodistribution of IgG2a or IgG1 monoclonal antibodies, suggesting that the response in rats was mainly against the IgG2b isotype.

In the clinical situation it is clear that not all patients produce significant levels of HAMA. In some patients the levels of HAMA are sufficient to affect the biodistribution of further imaging doses of antibody after only a single investigation. In others a number of repeat imaging investigations are possible without an apparent affect. However, it is surprising that even in inbred Wistar rats, of identical genetic background, age, and sex, and housed identically, that similar widespread variation of responses occurred following administration of antibody.

Using this model, the authors have shown that the generation of an antibody response correlates well with the incidence and magnitude of the perturbation and hepatic uptake of subsequent doses of radiolabelled antibody. The production of AMA titres of between $1/100$ and $1/78,000$ has been shown to cause equal effects on the altered biodistribution, although below $1/100$ the effect was more variable. No difference in the degree of the response has been demonstrated in this model when comparing antibody preparations radiolabelled with iodine to those radiolabelled with indium chelates.

Further studies examining the effect of the route of administration have also produced clinically relevant information. In particular, it has been observed that an intradermal injection of antibody was more immunogenic than the same dose given either intravenously or intraperitoneally. Furthermore, the administration of $\frac{1}{10}$th of the intravenous dose of antibody (often given clinically as skin test) given in addition to the intravenous dose significantly increases the resultant immune response rate compared to subjects receiving only the intravenous dose.

Further work has been carried out to investigate the effects of anti-idiotypic AMA in syngeneic BALB/c mice (Pimm et al., 1989). Anti-idiotypic AMA may be generated in this mouse model by the injection of 791T/36-ricin immunotoxin conjugate. The biodistribution of a subsequent dose of the same antibody showed increased hepatic clearance, indicating that anti-idiotypic antibodies alone may affect the biodistribution of repeat doses. To determine whether anti-idiotypic AMA could prevent localisation of antibody in tumours, serum from mice with anti-idiotypic AMA was injected into nude mice with human tumour xenografts. In these mice localisation of radiolabelled 791T/36 antibody was severely restricted.

Overall, these and similar studies provide information relevant to the design of antibody preparations suitable for clinical administration. The results with anti-idiotypic AMA are especially interesting, since attempts are currently being made to produce human or humanised (chimeric) antibodies to minimise the problems of the AMA response. In the light of these experimental findings, it would appear that the anti-idiotypic response will still present a clinical problem for the repeated administration of monoclonal antibody. These findings will need to be taken into account during the production of clinical protocols for both the diagnostic and therapeutic application of monoclonal antibodies.

POSSIBILITY OF HYPERSENSITIVE REACTIONS

Although the major problem with the production of HAMA is the formation of circulating immune complexes, resulting in deposition of the injected antibody in the liver and spleen and a reduction in image quality, there is also the possibility of the development of hypersensitive reactions. These reactions could be potentially hazardous to the patient. Although these reactions have only been rarely reported, investigators using monoclonal antibodies in immunoscintigraphy should be aware of their possible occurrence.

Hypersensitive reactions may be classified into five main types according to the speed of the reaction and the immune process involved. Clinically they will occur as a combination of symptoms and may not fit into one particular type.

Type I: Immediate Hypersensitivity

Type I hypersensitivity is a potentially serious reaction which occurs within minutes of exposure to the antigen and, if it was to occur, would normally be experienced immediately after intravenous injection of the imaging dose of antibody. This type of reaction would commonly be referred to as an anaphylactic reaction. It results from activation of mast cells which have bound IgE antibodies to their surface Fc receptors which, when they react with antigen (in this case the monoclonal antibody), causes them to degranulate and release vasoactive amines and spasmogens which cause smooth muscle contraction, increased vascular permeability, and a fall in blood pressure which may result in respiratory failure. The initial symptoms are of malaise and nausea, with a metallic taste in the mouth. These are rapidly followed by bronchoconstriction and circulatory collapse. If symptoms are severe and the patient experiences loss of pulse and respiration, treatment should be initiated with intravenous adrenaline. Similar Type I allergic reactions may occur in cases of acute inflammation, asthma, hay fever, and eczema.

Type II: Antibody-Mediated Hypersensitivity

Type II hypersensitive reactions are caused by the formation of antibody directed against cell surface antigens. In such reactions the cells become sensitised, leading to their destruction by cell-mediated cytotoxicity involving K cells or complement-mediated lysis. These type of reactions are responsible for the destruction of red cells following unmatched blood transfusions and haemolytic disease in the newborn.

Type III: Immune Complex Mediated Hypersensitivity

The formation of immune complexes of antibody and anti-antibody within the circulation may not result in any immediate clinical symptoms. In fact the only observable effects may be those visualised by immunoscintigraphy. As we have already seen, the formation of these complexes following administration of an imaging dose of antibody may have a dramatic effect on the biodistribution visualised by the gamma camera. The antibody complexes are cleared from the circulation by the cells of the reticuloendothelial system and may also be deposited in tissues and blood vessels. In severe instances the production of immune complexes will activate complement and attract polymorphs to the site of complex deposition, resulting in local damage. The production of immune complexes has been associated with various adverse reactions, including serum sickness and renal toxicity.

Type IV: Delayed Hypersensitivity

Delayed hypersensitivity occurs more than 12 hours following exposure to antigen. Local tissue damage may occur due to the attraction of macrophages by lymphokines released by antigen-sensitised T cells. This type of reaction is more commonly seen with skin contact and is the type more likely to be detected using a subcutaneous skin test dose of the antibody to be injected. However, the relatively long delay in the production of this reaction questions the use of the skin test as a screening method for patient compliance.

Type V: Stimulatory Hypersensitivity

This type of reaction is the least likely to be generated by the administration of monoclonal antibodies. In reactions of this kind, host tissue is stimulated by autoantibodies as a result of the immune system turning against the body's own tissues. Autoimmune disease occurs when autoantibodies result in pathological damage.

DETECTION OF ANTI-MOUSE ANTIBODY

In view of the importance of HAMA responses, it would be of great value to have simple methods for their detection. Patients could then be tested before the first and subsequent doses of monoclonal antibody. Ideally such a test should be able to give a clear guideline as to whether an investigation in an individual patient is likely to proceed without complications of either a clinical nature or in the performance of the imaging investigation. Early studies tended to use a skin test as a rough guide as to the possibility of hypersensitive reactions in patients. However, this method is unlikely to detect the presence of circulating HAMA, and now serum assays are being developed.

Skin Testing

In order to screen patients for potential anaphylactic reaction to an intravenous dose of monoclonal antibody, a subcutaneous or intradermal skin test has been advocated. This has normally consisted of 10% of the administered protein dose. A positive reaction in the form of a red flare occurring within 30 minutes of the test dose should certainly preclude patients from further doses of antibody.

Although this method should be able to detect immediate hypersensitivity reactions, the other type of response, including those of circulating HAMA, are not likely to be detected by this test. In general, experience has shown the skin test to be unreliable, and negative results were obtained in patients who were known to have circulating HAMA and in others in whom subsequent systemic hypersensitive reactions occurred. In addition, antibody is released slowly from the subcutaneous depot, thus further immunising the patient and increasing the likelihood of a reaction against further administered doses. Animal studies comparing intravenous, intradermal, and subcutaneous routes of administration with the production of AMA confirm this view (Durrant et al., 1989). Hence the use of the subcutaneous or intradermal skin test is considered to do more harm than good and should therefore be avoided.

Serum Assays

A variety of methods may be used for detecting the HAMA response in serum. These are radioimmunoassay, enzyme-linked immunoabsorbent assay, haemagglutination tests, and immunofluorescence tests. Because of the wide variation in normal individuals and the varying sensitivities of the different HAMA assays, it has been difficult to establish a normal range for a healthy population.

Serum from patients may be tested for HAMA by their ability to form immune complexes with the monoclonal antibody *in vitro*. This may be assessed by adding radiolabelled antibody, in the same form as that used for imaging to the serum. This should preferably be at the same concentration as that present *in vivo* immediately after intravenous injection. The formation of complexes may be detected by such procedures as size exclusion gel filtration on media such as Sephadex. This method has been used by, for example, Pimm et al. (1985) to show anti-mouse antibody responses in patients who have had repeated or even single doses of radiolabelled antibody for imaging (Fig. 6.6). This method has the advantage that it is detecting antibodies by complex formation in the same manner as they exert their effects *in vivo*. It also allows the ratio of radiolabelled antibody to serum to be varied, in keeping with the ratio of proposed dose to the calculated blood volume of the patient. This provides an estimate of the degree of complex formation which might be expected *in vivo* and allows some judgement of the clinical advisability of giving the patient the proposed dose of antibody. This method has the disadvantage, however, of being tedious and slow. It could be speeded up by the use of HPLC instead of conventional gel filtration, but that requires specialized apparatus and additional technical expertise.

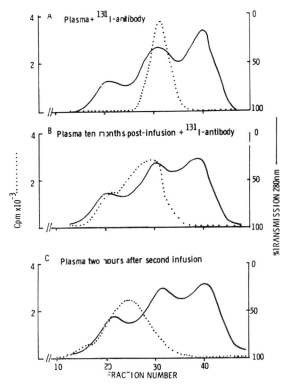

Fig. 6.6. Detection of HAMA by its ability to form immune complexes with radiolabelled monoclonal antibody. A: I-131 labelled 791T/36 monoclonal antibody was added to plasma from a patient with colo-rectal carcinoma who was to undergo immunoscintigraphy. The mixture of plasma and antibody was run on Sephacryl S300 gel filtration chromatography. The radiolabel elutes from the column as a distinct peak, coincident with the second peak of protein resulting from fractionation of the plasma proteins. B: Ten months after the patient's imaging investigation a plasma sample was taken, I-131 labelled antibody added and the chromatography repeated. There is a change in the elution profile of the radiolabel, part of it now running in a higher molecular size form, seen as a shift to earlier elution. This shows that the radiolabel present in the plasma is predominantly in the form of immune complexes formed by the patient's HAMA and the monoclonal antibody. C: The patient underwent a second injection of monoclonal antibody. Plasma taken two hours after this second injection was run on the chromatographic procedure, without the addition of further radiolabelled antibody. The radiolabelled monoclonal antibody in plasma is in high molecular size form, indicating that immune complexes had formed in vivo between the patient's HAMA and this second dose of radiolabelled monoclonal antibody. (Reproduced from Pimm et al., J. Nucl. Med. 26:1011–1023, 1985, with permission of the Society of Nuclear Medicine.)

As a consequence of the problems associated with the detection of anti-mouse antibody responses by demonstration of immune complex formation, other more widely used immunological techniques have been adapted to detect these types of anti-mouse antibody responses. Predominant among these have been ELISA assays. In these assays, target antigen, that is the mouse monoclonal antibody, is immobilized by adherence to the wells of microtitre plates, then exposed to the patient's serum, and the patient's antibody bound to the mouse monoclonal antibody is then detected with enzyme conjugated anti-human antiserum and an appropriate substrate for the enzyme. Serial dilutions of the serum can be tested and compared with results with control serum or serum from the patient before administration of the monoclonal antibody. The problem with this method is how to define positive reactions and, indeed, what exactly is meant by *positive*. Due to inter-test variations in absorbance values from ELISA assays, it is difficult to define an expected value for the control serum, such as a mean with standard deviations or two standard deviations outside of which a test sample could be considered to be statistically significantly different. Even if this could be done and the titre of a patient's serum could be said to be significantly raised over that expected from normal serum, it is not clear how this can be related to the possible *in vivo* consequences of giving that patient the monoclonal antibody in question. That is, how can we relate the titre *in vitro* of the patient's anti-mouse antibody response, detected by methods such as ELISA assays, to the ability of that antibody to perturb the biodistribution of monoclonal antibody if it was given intravenously? A "positive" control serum from a patient or sera from a number of patients in whom it was known that the biodistribution of the mouse monoclonal antibody had been affected could be included in each test if these were available in sufficient quantity, but even then one could not be sure that these only had the minimum amount of antibody to form complexes *in vivo* so that their ELISA values could be regarded as the maximum acceptable for serum from a patient to whom it was proposed to give the monoclonal antibody in question. Clearly there are a number of other problems with this approach. For example, the "positive" control serum should have come from patient(s) given the same antibody as it is proposed to give the patient whose serum is under test, since there are differences, both qualitative and quantitative, in the immunoge-

nicity of different monoclonal antibodies. Furthermore, the comparison in this sort of way of a "known positive" serum with that from a patient proposed to have a further dose of even the same monoclonal antibody would probably only be valid if the dose of monoclonal antibody for the proposed patient is the same as that which had been given to the "positive patient" when deleterious effects in its biodistribution had been seen.

A further problem in such assays for anti-mouse antibody is the choice of target monoclonal antibody. For example, if the target mouse antibody in the ELISA is a monoclonal antibody, it will be of only one isotype, but patients' responses, while including antibodies to the mouse immunoglobulin framework which would be detected in such an ELISA assay, will also include responses against the isotype administered. If the target monoclonal antibody in the ELISA is of a different isotype from that to which the patient has been exposed, then not all of the response can be detected. This problem could be overcome by using a mixture of monoclonal antibody isotypes as the target in the ELISA. But even then, anti-idiotypic responses, also frequently a major component of patients' immune responses to monoclonal antibodies, would not be detected. The ideal ELISA assay should have as its target monoclonal antibody the same one as the patient has been exposed to, or, to be more appropriate, that which it is proposed to give the patient. Thus, ideally an assay is needed for each individual monoclonal antibody.

Clearly there is a need for further development of rapid assays for anti-mouse antibodies in serum of patients to whom it is proposed to give repeated injections of mouse monoclonal antibodies. Kits for ELISA assays for anti-mouse antibody responses are now becoming available commercially from at least two companies, but due to the major anti-isotypic and anti-idiotypic components of patients' responses, these are unlikely to detect the full extent of a patient's response. Even ELISA assays can take several hours to run, and other well known techniques for antibody assays, such as agglutination of monoclonal antibody coated latex particles or red blood cells, warrant investigation as possibly more rapid assays which can be carried out while the patient waits in the clinic. But even if these assays can be set up, preferably for each individual monoclonal antibody, there remains the ability to be able to correlate the titre from these assays with the probable immunological and clinical consequences of the presence of these antibodies.

PREVENTION OF ANTI-MOUSE ANTIBODY RESPONSES

A number of manoeuvres have been suggested to overcome or avoid the problem of the immunogenicity of monoclonal antibodies, although as yet none can be regarded as consistently effective, and some are only at the stage of evaluation in animal models. As a result, the immune response remains a problem for multiple repeat investigations and may represent one of the major limitations of the technique.

Antibody Quality

It has been known for many years that the extent and nature of immune responses to purified proteins such as immunoglobulins in animals can depend on the quality of the preparation. Highly purified immunoglobulin, containing no aggregated material, when given by intravenous injection, will generally be poorly immunogenic compared with preparations containing aggregated material given by the same

route. Ledermann et al. (1988) have shown recently that in rabbits a monoclonal antibody preparation of clinical grade was less immunogenic after intravenous injection if aggregates had been removed by ultracentrifugation. It is important, therefore, that monoclonal antibody preparations for immunoscintigraphy are free of aggregated antibody. The purification stages of antibody production generally contain high speed centrifugation (usually at 50,000 to 100,000 $\times$ g for one hour) to remove damaged and aggregated antibody. But, of course, if the antibody is not stored correctly, is roughly handled, or is exposed to harsh conditions during labelling, aggregates may form again and contribute significantly to the immunogenicity of the preparation.

Protein Dose and Route of Injection

Although there is little data on the relative immunogenicity of different administered amounts of monoclonal antibody for immunoscintigraphy, it is probable that high doses would more immunogenic than lower doses. Many reported imaging investigations have used doses of up to a milligram or so of the monoclonal antibody. As discussed elsewhere, there is evidence with some antibodies that image sensitivity is dose-dependent, and there is perhaps the need to use higher doses, although how this influences immune response is at present unresolved.

The route of injection of monoclonal antibody will also be expected to influence its immunogenicity. It would be expected from past experiences with other purified proteins that intravenous injection would be the least immunogenic. Thus, when a particular monoclonal antibody proven not to be significantly immunogenic when given intravenously is given by another route (such as by intraperitoneal injection), it is possible that immune responses may become a problem. Classical immunological teaching states that to deliberately produce the greatest immune response an antigen should be given in an insoluble form and/or by a route which will produce a lasting depot of material. Thus any such injection—for example, a subcutaneous injection for lymphoscintigraphy—would be expected to be more immunogenic than an intravenous injection. As discussed elsewhere, an intradermal injection of monoclonal antibody to test for hypersensitivity may be produce a greater immune response than the subsequent intravenous dose for imaging.

It is apparent that different monoclonal antibodies, antibody fragments, and perhaps different isotypes of immunoglobulin, have different degrees of immunogenicity, although there is no hard data available on this. It may be that with those antibodies for which circulating antigens are present, the formation and clearance of immune complexes may increase the immunogenicity of the monoclonal antibody. Further experimental studies will be necessary before these aspects are understood.

Antibody Fragments

Fragments of antibody would be expected to be less immunogenic than complete antibody. The Fc portion of the molecule contains relatively large immunogenic regions, and its absence would therefore be expected to reduce the available antigenic sites against which an immune response may be generated. In addition, the biological handling of fragments is known to be different, and interactions with Fc receptors in the reticuloendothelial system, which would otherwise facilitate immune recognition, will be avoided. Unfortunately there is no complete answer to this problem. There is little data comparing patient responses to antibody with those of fragments of the same antibody when both have been given in identical doses and schedules. It is evident, however, that antibody responses are often still seen in patients given only antibody fragments. Moreover, with some antibodies it is difficult to make fragments, and in some imaging investigations it may be preferable to use intact antibody to avoid the high levels of radiolabel in the kidneys and bladder, which are generally seen with fragments.

Immunosuppression

One way to reduce the immune response to administered monoclonal antibody would be to give the patient some immunosuppressive treatment at the same time as the imaging dose. Previous experience with immunosuppressive agents such as steroids, azathioprine, and cyclophosphamide administered to patients receiving monoclonal antibodies for purposes other than immunoscintigraphy have not shown consistent benefit. Ledermann et al. (1988) have shown in a group of three patients with gastrointestinal tumours, each given four doses of 5 to 7 mg of an anti-CEA monoclonal antibody at two week intervals, that the immunosuppressive drug Cyclosporin A virtually abolished their immune response to the antibody. In this case the drug had been given orally for six days, starting two days before antibody administration, and all patients experienced side effects of nausea and anorexia.

If immunosuppressive treatment is to be successful in preventing sensitization of the patient to the monoclonal antibody, its value has to be balanced against the possible side effects of such immunosuppressive treatment. Such immunosuppression may perhaps be appropriate in a therapeutic situation—for example, in hospitalized cancer patients to be given multiple high doses of monoclonal antibodies conjugated to drugs or radionuclides. But it might not be appropriate, or logistically feasible, for cardiovascular imaging or for routine screening of patients for tumour recurrence.

Specific Abrogation

Another possible method of avoiding immune responses to monoclonal antibodies, which might be appropriate and feasible routinely, is a specific abrogation of the response to a particular monoclonal antibody. The immune response to an antigen, such as monoclonal antibody, involves the activation of B lymphocytes, which have the pre-determined ability to respond to that particular antigen in a subsequent encounter. These B lymphocytes take up the antigen onto their surface, then internalise and process it. Based on these considerations, if the antibody has a cytotoxic drug conjugated to it, the B lymphocytes may be killed following internalisation of the drug antibody conjugate. This would not only stop the current generation of antibody against the monoclonal antibody but leave the immune system permanently deficient in responsiveness to the particular monoclonal antibody. Different drugs, with different methods of linkage to the antibody, can be expected to have greater or lesser efficiencies for this effect. Using this approach, Durrant et al. (1989) have shown that a monoclonal antibody conjugated to the drug daunomycin did not induce antibody response in rats, whereas the untreated antibody did. It is significant that these rats failed to produce an immune response to several further doses of the antibody itself, and although they did eventually produce a response, it was much lower than that in untreated rats. This type of specific abrogation of responses to monoclo-

nal antibodies would be particularly attractive for clinical use, because only a single treatment might be necessary, which could be given at the same time as the imaging dose of monoclonal antibody. The specific nature of the suppression leaves other immune response of the patient unimpaired, and although a cytotoxic drug is conjugated to the monoclonal antibody, the dose is minute compared with that which might otherwise be used.

Human Monoclonal Antibodies

One of the main reasons for the current attempt to generate human monoclonal antibodies is the hope that they will be non-immunogenic in patients when given for imaging or therapeutic purposes. An alternative approach is to genetically engineer chimeric monoclonal antibodies in which the hypervariable region of a mouse monoclonal antibody, which contains the antigen recognition site, is incorporated into a human immunoglobulin (Colcher et al., 1989). Opinion is divided as to whether it is likely that anti-idiotypic responses will be generated to these human or humanized antibodies following administration to patients. Because clinical evaluation of these monoclonal antibodies is only just starting, there is little data available. Hale et al. (1988) have found that two patients given daily injections of up to 20 mg of a human-rat chimeric monoclonal antibody for therapy of lymphoma had no detectable antibody responses.

Even if anti-idiotypic responses are produced by patients in response to these monoclonal antibodies, it is not clear what effect they will have on their biodistribution and target localization. The authors have shown in model studies in mice that an antibody response restricted to the idiotope of a mouse monoclonal antibody can affect its biodistribution, with clearance to the liver and spleen. It is possible that some immune complexes formed between anti-idiotypic antibody and a monoclonal antibody may survive in the circulation rather than being cleared, although whether the monoclonal antibody with its combining site blocked by the anti-idiotypic antibody could still recognize antigen is uncertain.

REFERENCES AND FURTHER READING

Castello, G., Mansi, L., Leonardi, E., Lastoria, S., Melillo, G. (1988): Short term effects of i.v. injected murine Tc-99m-F(ab')$_2$ fragments of an anti-melanoma antibody (HMW-MAA 225.28s) on haemato-immunological parameters in patients with melanoma. Int. J. Biol. Markers 3:140–144.

Colcher, D., Milenic, D., Roselli, M., Rabitschek, A., Yarranton, G., King, D., Adais, J., Whittle, N., Bodmer, M., Schlom, J. (1989): Characterization and biodistribution of recombinant and recombinant/chimeric constructs of monoclonal antibody B72:3. Cancer Res. 49:1738–1745.

Courtenay-Luck, N.S., Epenetos, A.A., Moore, R., Larche, M., Pectasides, D., Dhokia, B., Ritter, M.A. (1986): Development of primary and secondary immune responses to mouse monoclonal antibodies used in the diagnosis and therapy of malignant neoplasms. Cancer Res. 46:6489–6493.

Durrant, L.D., Robins, R.A., Marksman, R.A., Garnett, M.C., Ogunmuyiwa, Y., Baldwin, R.W. (1989): Abrogation of antibody responses in rats to murine monoclonal antibody 791T/36 by treatment with daunomycin-cis-aconityl-791T/36 conjugates. Cancer Immunol. Immunother. 28:37–42.

Ford, E.H., Lee, R.E., Sharkey, R.M., Alger, E.A., Horowitz, J.A., Hall, T.C., Goldenberg, D.M. (1988): Effect of human anti-mouse antibody (HAMA) on monoclonal antibody (Mab) biokinetics and biodistribution during a phase I/II radioimmunotherapy clinical trial. J. Nucl. Med. 29:761 (Abstract).

Hale, G., Dyer, M.J.S., Clark, M.R., Phillips, J.M., Marcus, R., Reichmann, L., Winter, G., Waldmann, H. (1988): Remission induction in non-Hodgkin Lymphoma with reshaped human monoclonal antibody CAMPATH-1H. Lancet 2:1394–1399.

Ledermann, J.A., Begent, R.H.J., Bagshawe, K.D. (1988): Cyclosporin A prevents the anti-murine antibody response to a monoclonal anti-tumour antibody in rabbits. Br. J. Cancer 58:562–566.

Ledermann, J.A., Begent, R.H.J., Bagshawe, K.D., Riggs, S.J., Searle, F., Glaser, M.G., Green, A.J., Dale, R.G. (1988): Repeated anti-tumour antibody therapy in man with suppression of the host response by Cyclosporin A. Br. J. Cancer 58: 654–657.

Perkins, A.C., Pimm, M.V., Powell, M.C. (1988): The implications of patient antibody response for the clinical usefulness of immunoscintigraphy. Nucl. Med. Comm. 9:273–282.

Pimm, M.V., Durrant, L.G., Baldwin, R.W. (1989): The influence of syngeneic anti-idiotypic antibody on the biodistribution of an anti-tumour monoclonal antibody in BALB/c mice. Int. J. Cancer 43:147–151.

Pimm, M.V., Perkins, A.C., Armitage, N.C., Baldwin, R.W. (1985): The characteristics of blood-borne radiolabels and the effect of anti-mouse IgG antibodies on localisation of radiolabelled monoclonal antibodies in cancer patients. J. Nucl. Med. 26: 1011–1023.

Pimm, M.V., Perkins, A.C., Durrant, L.G., Baldwin, R.W. (1988): A rat model for imaging the effect of anti-mouse antibody responses on the biodistribution of radiolabelled mouse monoclonal antibodies. Eur. J. Nucl. Med. 14:507–511.

Van Kroonenburgh, N.J.P.G., Pauwels, E.K.J. (1988): Human immunological response to mouse monoclonal antibodies in the treatment or diagnosis of malignant diseases. Nucl. Med. Commun. 9:919–930.

7 Clinical Role of Immunoscintigraphy

CLINICAL SCENARIO

A range of clinical investigations is often performed to obtain diagnostic information. Many of these procedures are invasive and carry inherent risks and morbidity. The majority of imaging techniques such as radiography, ultrasound, magnetic resonance, and radionuclide imaging are capable of outlining internal body anatomy with minimal patient trauma. The size of the smallest lesion which may be detected will depend upon the characteristics of the lesion which differ from those of normal tissue (for example density, chemical content, or the ability of the lesion to take up a tracer). Visualisation of the lesion is ultimately limited by the resolution of the imaging system, and it follows therefore that by the time a change in anatomy is observed the disease will be well advanced. One of the strengths of nuclear medicine is the ability of radiopharmaceuticals to trace abnormal physiology precursive to lesion formation. In some cases this provides diagnostic information unobtainable by any other imaging modality. For example, in bone imaging the alter-

ation in osteoblastic activity and blood supply occurs at an earlier stage than the change in density required to produce a radiographic change.

The most successful approach to radionuclide imaging is to use a particular characteristic of pathological tissue not found in normal tissues. Utilising such a property results in the concentration of a tracer at the lesion site, resulting in an area of increased uptake. The main properties exploited for this targeting approach are metabolism, blood supply, perfusion, and the presence of specific receptors or antigens. Such properties apply equally to targeting therapeutic agents as for diagnostic imaging. The specificity of the radiopharmaceutical is of fundamental importance since the ultimate contrast between the lesion and the surrounding tissues will determine the accuracy of lesion detection from the final images. With the exception of radioiodine and MIBG, most radiopharmaceuticals are not highly selective with respect to the tissues within which they concentrate. In oncology the physiological characteristics exploited for targeting conventional radiopharmaceuticals to tumour tissues have hitherto been largely non-specific. The use of antibodies and in particular monoclonal antibodies has heralded a new era in the localisation of tracers within pathological sites. Yet despite initial claims (mainly with the use of antibodies for tumour imaging), progress has been slow, and the use of monoclonal antibodies in routine clinical diagnosis is only now becoming a reality. Looking at the number of monoclonal antibodies which are now available (see Appendix: Antibody Look Up Table, this volume), one can see a vast range of materials offering clinical potential. These antibodies show a spread of reactivity from tumour-associated antigens, through cell specific antigens and metal chelates.

The application of monoclonal antibodies for radiolabelling circulating blood cells and serum proteins is perhaps the most exciting development in immunoscintigraphy. Following a simple intravenous injection of antibody it is now possible to radiolabel circulating cells such as platelets and granulocytes *in vivo*. This approach is revolutionising radiopharmacy practice. Previously, cell labelling techniques involved time-consuming procedures within the radiopharmacy for cell separation, incubation, resuspension, and washing, before re-injecting the final radiolabelled cells into the patient. Initially antibodies associated with blood cells were generated as a by-product of work carried out in the search for antibodies associated with tumour antigens. These antibodies were at first discarded by research workers since they were not associated with tumour antigens or exhibited unwanted cross-reactivity with normal tissues. Subsequently it was realised that these antibodies were of clinical value in nuclear medicine. More recently work has been carried out with the specific inten-

tion of producing antibodies for radiolabelling specific populations of cells or serum proteins. A broad range of antibodies now exist, and to date these have largely been of relevance in the detection of thromboembolism and abscess and inflammation.

From the large number of clinical trials that have been carried out in Western Europe and the United States, workers are now beginning to determine which antibodies are the most suitable for clinical use. The production of efficient and reliable radiolabelling techniques using radionuclides such as In-111, I-123, and Tc-99m have resulted in a range of products suitable for routine clinical application. Manufacturers are now considering the marketing implications, and the first product licences for immunoradiopharmaceuticals have now been granted. This chapter describes some of the main monoclonal antibody preparations that have been used for clinical imaging and examines their clinical role and diagnostic value.

IMMUNOSCINTIGRAPHY IN ONCOLOGY

The majority of antibody imaging work has previously concentrated on the detection of tumour deposits. This is mainly because the antibodies that were first produced were raised against antigens that were associated with tumours. Whilst in oncology therapeutic procedures still appear rather limited, there is now evidence of an expansion in the diagnostic application of monoclonal antibodies. The use of *in vitro* assays for monitoring the level of serum antigens and immunohistology for the classification of tissue sections is having a dramatic effect on departments of biochemistry and pathology. Some serum antigens which are now routinely assayed are given in Table 7.1. The use of such assays on a

TABLE 7.1. The Main Serum Tumour Antigens Monitored by Monoclonal Antibodies

Cancer type	Antigen
Colorectal	CEA
	19.9
	TAG 72
Ovary	CA125
	CA15.3
	PLAP
Breast	CA15.3
Oesophagus	SCCA
Cervix	SCCA
Testis	AFP
Hepatoma	AFP

serial basis will simply indicate the presence of increasing antigen levels in the circulation (reflecting tumour growth). These have been shown to be of greater use in the detection of secondary rather than primary cancer. Imaging studies are indicated in patients with abnormally raised serum antigen levels or in patients with other clinical indications of recurrent or metastatic spread of disease. The main areas of investigation continue to be in the detection of gastrointestinal and gynaecological cancer. It is interesting to note that not all tumour-associated antigens are shed into the blood stream, and some antibodies reacting with antigens fixed to cell surfaces look hopeful candidates for tumour imaging. The P72 glycoprotein associated with the 791T/36 antibody which has been used extensively by the authors is a typical example. As with most radionuclide imaging studies, immunoscintigraphy has a limited resolution. However, the technique does have the advantage of being able to detect tumour recurrence and distant me-

tastases with only one injection, and it may be especially useful in cases where CT and MRI are equivocal due to abnormal patient anatomy and tissue scarring following initial surgery.

Immunoscintigraphy of Gastrointestinal Cancer

Gastrointestinal malignancy is responsible for approximately 30% of all cancer-related deaths in the western world. Despite advances in the diagnosis and treatment of gastrointestinal malignancy, a large proportion of patients have extensive disease at the time of the initial diagnosis. Subsequently, a large proportion of patients ultimately die of recurrent or metastatic disease. The largest single cancer type in this group is colorectal cancer, which contributes one quarter of the deaths due to gastrointestinal malignancy. The main curative method is surgical resection, but additional therapeutic measures such as radiotherapy are often necessary since the disease is disseminated in about one quarter of patients referred. It is therefore apparent that there is considerable clinical pressure for the development of diagnostic techniques for the accurate detection and staging of gastrointestinal malignancy.

Anti-CEA antibodies. A great deal of effort was originally directed towards the identification of antigens specific for gastrointestinal cancers. It was subsequently realised that antigens present at low concentrations in normal tissues were sometimes elevated in certain cancers. In some cases these were shed into the circulation and could be detected by serum assays. The antigen first recognised as being associated with colorectal cancer was carcinoembryonic antigen (CEA), which was first described by Gold and Freedman in 1965. In 1978 the first successful clinical imaging of colorectal cancer was reported by

Goldenberg et al., using I-131-labelled hyperimmune goat antiserum prepared following immunisation with CEA. The use of this antiserum to image other GI malignancies such as stomach and pancreas was less successful. Studies followed by other centres using other polyclonal anti-CEA antibodies radiolabelled with I-131. The first use of a monoclonal anti-CEA antibody was reported by Mach et al. in 1981.

Antibodies raised against CEA have been used more than antibodies of any other type. Hence they are generally considered the most valuable antibodies for imaging colorectal cancer at the present time. The antibodies which have received the most clinical attention include C46 (IgG2a), ZCE-025 (IgG1), F023C5 (IgG1), and BW431/26 (IgG1). In general, immunoscintigraphy using anti-CEA antibodies has resulted in sensitivies greater than 80% (Goldenberg, 1978; Dykes et al., 1980; Armitage et al., 1986; Begent et al., 1986; Delaloye et al., 1986). For comparison, the results taken from a selection of published studies using various antibodies are shown in Table 7.2. These results should only be used as a broad guide for the capabilities of the technique in the detection of GI tumours. Comparisons of published data is problematical, and direct parallels cannot be drawn since the patient groups varied greatly. Furthermore, some of these studies are retrospective, whereas other studies give a prospective evaluation of the antibody, the latter being more clinically relevant. A prospective trial comprising In-111-C46 anti-CEA antibody with magnetic resonance imaging (0.15 Tesla) and X-ray CT has been carried out in Nottingham. This study was carried out by imaging 35 patients attending a colorectal cancer clinic who had previously had a resection for carcinoma of the colon or rectum. The results are given in Table 7.3. Few comparative studies of this nature

have previously been undertaken; however, carefully controlled prospective evaluations of this nature are essential if the clinical value of immunoscintigraphy is to be determined. Figure 7.1 shows examples of a patient with recurrent colorectal cancer imaged with all three modalities. Figure 7.2 shows an example of a patient with tumour recurrence in whom X-ray CT and MRI were found to be normal.

The choice of radiolabel, antibody fragment, and imaging technique are obviously important, and it is to be expected that observer experience is also a critical factor in the performance of published studies. The visualisation of tumours will clearly be improved if antibodies with higher tumour-to-no-tumour ratios are developed. T:NT ratios of around 3:1 have commonly been reported (Mach et al., 1981). Since the early 1980s steady progress has been made using monoclonal anti-CEA antibodies and especially with the technology associated with radiolabelling, first with the use of I-123 anti-CEA antibody (Delaloye et al., 1986), then with the production of an In-111-labelled high-affinity monoclonal antibody to CEA (C46, Armitage et al., 1986), and more recently with the BW 431/26 antibody which was radiolabelled with Tc-99m (Baum et al., 1989). The development of an efficient Tc-99m-labelled preparation which could be used routinely heralded a new era in immunoscintigraphy. An image of a patient with colonic cancer using Tc-99m-BW431/26 antibody is given in Figure 7.3. When compared with In-111-anti-CEA antibodies, Tc-99m-labelling appears to result in a reduction in the accumulation of tracer in normal liver. It is anticipated that Tc-99m-labelling will result in an improvement in the rate of detection of liver metastases. The high uptake of In-111-labelled antibodies by the reticuloendothelial system and in particular the liver has resulted in an extremely

TABLE 7.2. Detection of Gastrointestinal Cancer by Immunoscintigraphy

Antibody	Radiolabel	Tumours (number)	Sensitivity of detection (%)	Reference
Polyclonal CEA intact	I-131	P (5) S (11)	80 73	Dykes et al., 1980
Polyclonal CEA intact	I-131	P (7) S (25)	100 80	Kim et al., 1980
Polyclonal CEA intact	I-131	P (12) S (53)	83 92	Goldenberg et al., 1983
Polyclonal CEA intact	I-131	S (31)	94	Begent et al., 1986
Monoclonal CEA C46 intact	In-111	P (7) S (11)	100 72	Armitage et al., 1986
Monoclonal CEA F(ab')$_2$	I-123	P (4) S (13)	100 77	Delaloye et al., 1986
Monoclonal CEA Fab	I-123	P (6) S (21)	100 86	Delaloye et al., 1986
Monoclonal 17-1A	I-131	Mixed	59	Chatal et al., 1984
Monoclonal 19-9	I-131	Mixed	66	
Monoclonal CEA + 19-9 F(ab')$_2$	I-131	Mixed	77	Chatal et al., 1984
Monoclonal 791T/36 intact	I-131	Mixed	90	Farrands et al., 1982
Monoclonal B72.3 intact	I-131	Mixed	70	Esteban et al., 1987
Monoclonal CEA (ZCE 025 intact)	In-111	Mixed	90	Abel-Nabi et al., 1987
Monoclonal CEA (BW431/26 intact)	Tc-99m	Mixed	91	Baum et al., 1989
Monoclonal CEA (C46 intact)	In-111	Mixed	95	Granowska et al., 1989

P = Primary tumour.
S = Secondary tumour.

TABLE 7.3. A Comparison of Immunoscintigraphy MRI and X-Ray CT in the Detection of Pelvic Recurrence Following Resection of Colorectal Carcinoma

	0.15T MRI	In-111-C46 anti-CEA	X-ray CT
	n = 33	n = 23	n = 32
Sensitivity %	84	85	94
Specificity %	46	60	63
Positive predictive value %	70	73	71
Negative predictive value %	67	75	91

poor performance for the detection of liver metastases. However, one of the strengths of immunoscintigraphy is its ability to detect distant metastases following only one injection of antibody. Figure 7.4 shows an example of tomographic imaging with an anti-CEA antibody (In-111-228), showing uniform high uptake in liver and metastases in the chest. Tomography has been found to be of particular value in such cases (Perkins et al., 1988).

In routine clinical practice elevated serum levels of CEA provide a valuable indication for imaging (Begent et al., 1986). Studies carried out by Kim et al. (1980) have shown that circulating serum levels of CEA as high as 5,600 ng/ml did not interfere with the successful imaging of colorectal tumours. Immunoscintigraphy is considered to be especially helpful in the follow-up of patients who have had initial curative surgery for the resection of a primary tumour. In these patients other diagnostic imaging modalities such as X-ray CT and MRI may be difficult to interpret because of the altered abdomino-pelvic anatomy resulting from previous surgery. In cases where CT and MRI are equivocal, immunoscintigraphy is the next investigation of choice.

19.9 Antibody. The monoclonal antibody 116 NS 19.9 reacts with a carbohydrate antigenic determinant (sialylated lacto-N-fucopentaose II) CA19.9. This antigen has been found at low concentrations in the sera from healthy individuals but is frequently increased in sera from patients with adenocarcinomas. Imaging studies using intact or $F(ab')_2$ fragments of this antibody radiolabelled with I-131 showed significant accumulation in 19 out of 29 sites (66%) of colorectal cancer (Chatal et al., 1984). However, this antibody appears to be of greater value for the detection of small intestinal tumours and, in particular, tumours of the pancreas. Chatal et al. (1984) reported 100% positive immunohistochemical staining of 23 adenocarcinomas of the pancreas, stomach, and biliary tract with 19.9 antibody, whereas reaction with anti-CEA antibody was positive on 78% (18 of 23) of sections. For comparison, immunohistological staining of 36 colorectal adenocarcinomas was positive in 81% cases using 19.9 antibody and 94% using anti-CEA antibody. The higher specificity of 19.9 for gastric and small bowel tumours has led to the production of a 19.9 anti-CEA antibody cocktail (Chatal et al., 1984). However, the use of such cocktails merely broadens the sensitivity of the imaging preparation and has not been widely adopted for diagnosis. The use of an antibody cocktail would appear more favourable for therapy because of the heterogeneity of tumour antigen expression.

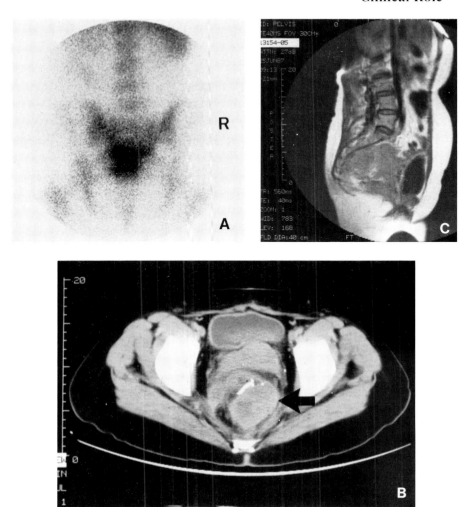

Fig. 7.1. Comparative imaging of a 52-year-old female patient with a proven recurrence of carcinoma of the rectum. A: Posterior immunoscintigraphy of the pelvis 72 hours after administration of 1 mg (80 MBq/2 mCi) of In-111-C46 anti-CEA antibody. B: CT image showing tumour mass (arrow) with suture clip remaining from initial surgery. C: Sagittal SE 560/40 (T_1 weighted) MRI image showing the large posterior mass. (Unpublished studies carried out at University Hospital, Nottingham.)

791T/36 Antibody. There have been a number of antibodies raised against tumours not of gastrointestinal origin that have proven to be of value for imaging colorectal tumours. In Nottingham the monoclonal antibody 791T/36, (IgG2b) originally raised against a human osteosarcoma cell line has been successfully used to detect colorectal tumours. Specific localisation has been demonstrated since the 72,000 dalton glycoprotein antigen defined by the 791T/36 antibody has been isolated from colorectal tumour cells (Price et al., 1984). However, this antigen has not been detected in the circulation of patients with colorectal cancer. The assay

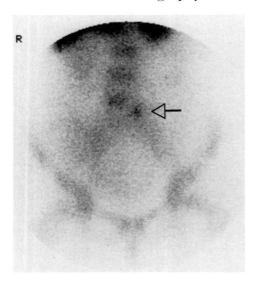

Fig. 7.2. Anterior image of the lower abdomen of a 49-year-old female patient 9 months following surgical resection of a recto-sigmoid carcinoma. Uptake of In-111-C46 anti-CEA antibody 48 hours after administration of 1 mg (80 MBq/2 mCi) is visible to the left of the lower lumbar vertebra. This recurrence was missed by CT scan and MRI and confirmed at laparotomy.

of resected specimens from patients with colorectal cancer injected with I-131-791T/36 and I-123 irrelevant IgG has shown that this antibody was taken up with a tumour-to-normal-colon ratio of the order of 2.5:1 (Armitage et al., 1984).

The use of Fab fragments of 791T/36 have not shown specific tumour localisation, and *in vitro* tests have shown that the fragments have a low binding capacity. To date it has not been possible to produce F(ab′)$_2$ fragments of 791T/36, and hence clinical studies have been carried out using intact antibody. Radiolabelling with either I-131 or In-111 has enabled imaging of both primary and disseminated disease (Armitage et al., 1984, 1985). In particular, the use of In-111 as the radiolabel improved the performance of the imaging technique and permitted high quality imaging by emission tomography. Use of

this antibody may prove to be of value in patients with a suspicion of recurrent cancer following previous surgical resection of the primary tumour.

A prospective study carried out in 23 patients with a clinical suspicion of abdominal and/or pelvic recurrence using In-111-labelled 791T/36 antibody has been undertaken. The results showed that immunoscintigraphy was capable of providing clinically useful information, especially where CT scanning revealed an anatomical abnormality which was not clearly indicative of recurrent disease. Positive immunoscintigraphy in such cases can confirm the presence of recurrent tumour and differentiate lesions from inflammatory masses.

Other antibodies. The B72.3 antibody (IgG1) was raised against a membrane-enriched fraction of a human carcinoma. It recognises a high-molecular-weight tumour-associated glycoprotein (TAG-72) which is expressed in approximately 90% of colorectal carcinomas but also reacts with 85% of breast carcinomas and 95% of ovarian carcinomas. The TAG-72 antigen detected by the B72.3 antibody has been shown to be secreted by tumour cells and can be found in the circulation of some patients with colorectal cancer.

Imaging studies in 27 patients using I-131-labelled B72.3 antibody were reported by Colcher et al. (1987), who noted that 52% of tumour deposits were correctly detected. The use of alternative radiolabels may improve the initially low reported result.

Another of the more recently developed antibodies is the antibody PRIA3. This is directed against a columnar cell surface antigen. Granowska et al. (1989) have used the technique of Schwarz (1987) for Tc-99m radiolabelling the PRIA3 monoclonal antibody. Thirteen patients were imaged using Tc-99m PRIA3 at 10 min, 2, 4, 6, and 24 h with tomography at 5 h. High

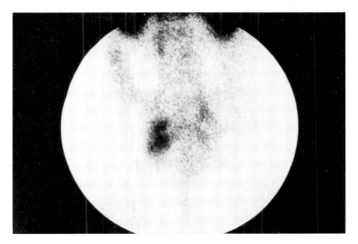

Fig. 7.3. Posterior image of the pelvis of patient 4 hours after injection of 2 mg (1.1 GBq 30 mCi of Tc-99m– BW431/26 anti-CEA antibody. Clear visualisation of a pelvic recurrence and suspicion of para-aortic lymph node metastases were seen 8 months after resection of a sigmoid colon cancer. Serum CEA levels were elevated for several months (17.2 μg/ml). Repeat CT scans, ultrasound and colonoscopy were normal. Subsequently the immunoscintigraphy findings were confirmed histologically and by immunohistochemistry. (Study provided by Dr. R.P. Baum Assistant Professor of Nuclear Medicine, University Hospital, Frankfurt, FRG.)

quality images with positive tumour identification as early as 4 h were achieved. The blood clearance half-life was 24 h for the slow phase with 12% of the injected activity excreted in the urine per day. No unblocked thyroid uptake was seen at 24 h, confirming *in vivo* stability. There were 11 positive images: 9/9 primary, one pelvic recurrence, and one recurrent villous adenoma; and two normal images, mild inflammatory bowel disease and one possible recurrence confirmed as true negative by tissue biopsy. This work demonstrated that Tc-99m PRIA3 would be acceptable for the routine detection of colorectal cancer.

Immunoscintigraphy of Gynaecological Cancer

Monoclonal antibodies are now an established method for the detection of tumour recurrence in patients with gynaecological malignancy. The assay of tumour markers, mainly CA125, has given the clini-

cian a means for monitoring patients following surgery. Imaging studies are also providing of value in the follow-up of these patients. A review of the present state of the art of immunoscintigraphy in the detection of ovarian carcinoma is a task fraught with difficulty. From the literature which has hitherto appeared on the monoclonal antibodies employed in clinical imaging trials, HMFG1/2, OC125, H317, H17E2, NDOG2, and 791T/36 are the main antibodies which have been used. A comparison of the performance of immunoscintigraphy from selected published studies is given in Table 7.4. The main conclusion that is reached is that no one of these antibodies is clearly superior to any other *in vivo* and that immunoscintigraphy cannot totally replace laparotomy for diagnosing ovarian cancer at the present time. The main role for the technique is in the follow-up of ovarian cancer and monitoring therapeutic response.

As with colorectal cancer, relatively high sensitivity of tumour detection above

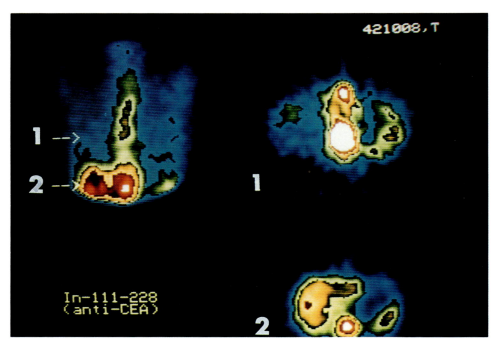

Fig. 7.4. Images of a patient with bone metastases from colon carcinoma imaged 48 hours following injection of 1 mg (80 MBq/2 mCi) In-111-228 antibody. **Left:** Anterior planar view of the thorax showing the position of the axial slices 1 and 2. (Abnormal uptake is poorly visualised in this view due to the high uptake in the liver). **Top Right:** Axial reconstructed SPECT view showing normal uptake in bone marrow (spine and sternum) and abnormal uptake in the ribs (seen mainly on the left side of the patient). **Bottom Right:** Axial slice showing normal distribution of activity in the liver, spleen and spine.

80% sensitivity has generally been reported. Other imaging modalities such as X-ray CT and MRI and ultrasound have not been previously shown to have a dramatic impact on the management of patients with recurrent gynaecological disease. Thus immunoscintigraphy offers more to this group of patients than many of the others with malignant disease. The use of the technique as an alternative to second-look surgery has been widely suggested (Symonds et al., 1985). However, Epenetos et al. (1985) using antibodies associated with PLAP (H317 and H17E2) came to the conclusion that positive antibody imaging indicates the definite presence of tumour, although negative imaging does not always exclude the presence of disease.

The most valuable of clinical trials are those carried out prospectively. Powell et al. (1987) carried out an assessment of the 791T/36 antibody in 123 patients with suspected primary or recurrent gynaecological cancer. The relative sensitivity and specificity of detection of tumours of ovary, cervix, and corpus are given in Table 7.5. Such studies show the diagnostic capabilities of the technique, but the specificity of tumour detection using monoclonal antibodies is still in question. Evaluation of immunoscintigraphy should not be carried out in isolation from other radiological modalities. Perkins et al. (1990) carried out a pilot study to compare immunoscintigraphy using I-131-OC125 F(ab')$_2$ and magnetic resonance imaging in patients with ovarian cancer. (An example of

TABLE 7.4. Clinical Studies of Immunoscintigraphy in Ovarian Cancer

Antibody	Label	Patients	Sens (%)	Spec (%)	Reference
NDOG2	I-123	15	84	50	Davies et al., 1985
HMFG2	I-123	9	89	—	Epenetos et al., 1982
		40	92	—	Granowska et al., 1984
		25	89	83	Patiesky et al., 1985
791T/36	In-111 I-131	30 Primary	100	69	Powell et al., 1987
		48 Recurrent	96	86	
OC-125	I-131	13 Primary	100	33	Barzen et al., 1989
		30 Recurrent	86	75	

subtraction imaging using I-131-OC125 is given in Fig. 5.2, Chapter 5, this volume.) This study concluded that MRI was superior in the detection of small tumour deposits (of <1 cm diameter) but that immunoscintigraphy was better suited in the assessment of widespread and metastatic disease. Imaging using In-111-OC125 antibody has shown to be of greater clinical value because of the improved image quality when compared with I-131. This antibody has been advocated mainly for the detection of serous ovarian tumours, whereas 19.9 antibody is considered more suitable for the detection of mucinous tumours. An example comparing In-111-OC125 with MRI in a patient with a primary ovarian tumour is given in Figure 7.5.

Clinically, this technique is of value for the determination of malignant components of large cystic masses (Figure 7.6). However, occasionally misleading results may be obtained (Figure 7.7).

A prospective multi-centre evaluation of In-111-OC125 F(ab')$_2$ antibody has been carried out in Europe in conjunction with the International Research Group for Immunoscintigraphy and Immunotherapy (IRIST) and CIS International (Saclay, France). This study comprised 59 patients investigated at one of six centres (Aachen, Frankfurt, Nantes, Nottingham, Reims, and Rennes). All patients were in remission following previous surgery for removal of primary ovarian carcinoma. The results comparing immunoscintigraphy with X-ray CT

TABLE 7.5. Sensitivity and Specificity of Immunoscintigraphy Using 791T/36 Antibody in Gynaecological Cancer

Tumour	Number	Sensitivity (%)	Specificity (%)
Ovary	73	98	79
Cervix	20	65	100
Corpus	17	85	60
Recurrent disease	65	92	88

From Powell et al., 1987.

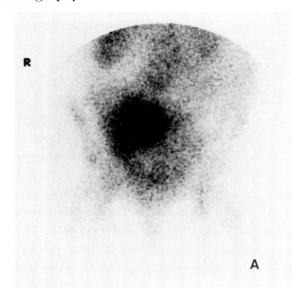

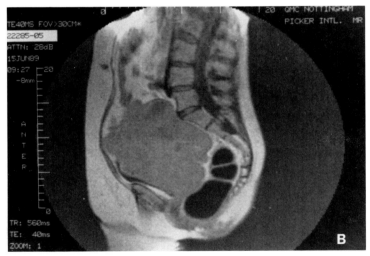

Fig. 7.5A,B

and abdominal ultrasound are given in Tables 7.6A, B and C.

Two new monoclonal antibodies which appear promising for the detection of gynaecological pathology have recently been developed. One such antibody OV-TL3 raised against ovarian cancer has a relatively high sensitivity for ovarian carcinomas, and its antigen is not shed into the circulation. Massuger et al. (1989) as-

sessed the safety and preliminary diagnostic accuracy of In-111-F(ab')$_2$ fragments in 15 patients who were imaged after i.v. administration of 140 MBq (3.8 mCi) In-111-OV-TL3 F(ab')$_2$. Planar and SPECT images were recorded at intervals between 4 and 96 hours after injection. In all patients CT scanning was performed and 10 patients were operated upon within a few days following immunoscintigraphy. Besides a

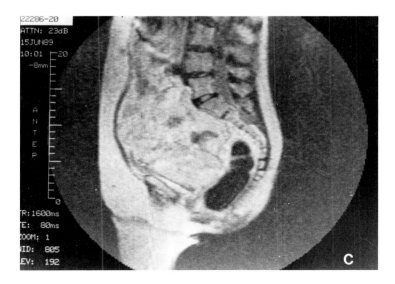

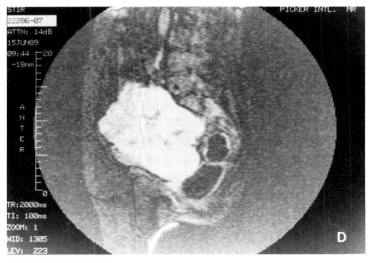

Fig. 7.5. A: Anterior view of the pelvis of a 76-year-old patient with a primary adenocarcinoma of the ovary 72 hours following injection of 80 MBq (2 mCi) In-111-OC125 antibody. Uptake in this large tumour mass can be clearly seen. B: SE 560/40 (T$_1$ weighted) image C: SE 1600/80 (T$_2$ weighted) image D: STIR sagittal MRI image through the same tumour mass. (Unpublished studies carried out at University Hospital, Nottingham.)

transient rash in one patient, no adverse reactions were observed. In the patients who underwent operation, excellent conformity was seen between scintigraphic and surgical results. Tumour uptake was between 0.1 and 5% of the administered dose. The total urinary excretion was approximately 17%, and total stool activity approximately 2% of the dose.

A further monoclonal antibody which has been characterised and found to be highly specific for human ovarian carcinoma is MOV18. This antibody has been shown to react with tissue sections of 79%

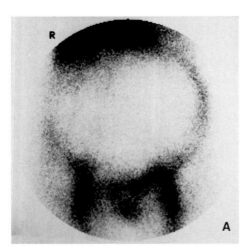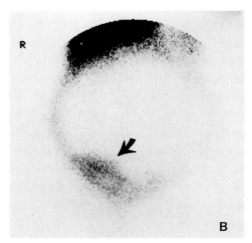

Fig. 7.6. Example showing the uptake of In-111-OC125 antibody in the solid malignant component of a large cystic tumour of the left ovary. Following surgery histology showed the mass to be a mucinous cystadenoma associated with a Brener tumour. **A:** Blood pool image. **B:** 72 hour image. (Unpublished studies carried out at University Hospital, Nottingham.)

of ovarian epithelial tumours and only 2% of a wide range of other epithelial tumours. No reactivity has been found on non-epithelial tumours, normal cells, and normal tissues. Buraggi et al. (1989) have carried out a clinical trial to study the biodistribution of this antibody and determine its clinical applications. Only patients with known ovarian carcinoma were considered. MOV18 labelled with I-131 was injected i.v. into 19 patients. Five additional patients underwent i.p. administration which was preceded by Tc-99m scan to check if peritoneal perfusion was adequate. Whole-body and regional scans were performed during the first 3 hours after the antibody injection and successively every 24 hours for about 1–2 weeks. After immunoscintigraphy all the patients underwent laparotomy and the immunoscintigraphic results were compared with the surgical findings. Laparotomy showed 44 abdominal and 28 pelvic lesions. Of the total of 72 major tumour sites, 52 (72%) were correctly detected by imaging. 89%

(25/28) of the pelvic lesions and 61% (27/44) of the abdominal sites were detected.

Second-look surgery is regarded as the most effective means of follow-up for the patient who has had previous surgery for gynaecological malignancy. A number of workers have examined the use of highly collimated surgical probes for detection of tumour deposits during operation. The use of such probes remains to be demonstrated as clinically beneficial in the assessment of these patients. Some workers have investigated alternative routes of administration in the assessment of ovarian cancer. In many respects this approach has been adopted because of the less than ideal specificity of antibodies that are currently available. Since ovarian cancer is largely restricted to the peritoneal cavity, it is postulated that this disease may be more effectively treated by intraperitoneal (IP) injection rather than systemic administration, and the group at the Hammersmith Hospital in London have investigated treatment of recurrent disease using I-131

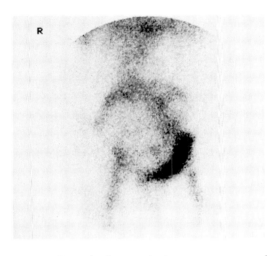

Fig. 7.7. Example showing the image appearance of In-111-OC125 antibody 72 hours after injection in a patient with a bulky mass which was subsequently found to be uterine fibroids. Intense uptake in the left side of the pelvis was due to the retention of a large volume of urine in the bladder.

and Y-90 labelled antibody. Perkins et al. (1989) combined an examination of the biokinetics and biodistribution of IP administered I-131 or In-111-labelled 791T/

TABLE 7.6A. Results of a European Multi-Centre Trial Comparing In-111-OC125 Immunoscintigraphy (I.S.) With C.T.

		I.S.		
C.T.	TP	TN	FP	FN
TP	15	—	—	1
TN	—	19	4	—
FP	—	6		—
FN	16	—	—	5
	I.S. 55/66		C.T 39/66	
Accuracy	(85%)		(59%)	
Sensitivity	(88%)		(43%)	
Specificity	(80%)		(79%)	

TABLE 7.6B. Results of a European Multi-Centre Trial Comparing In-111-OC125 Immunoscintigraphy (I.S.) With Ultrasound (U.S.)

		I.S.		
U.S.	TP	TN	FP	FN
TP	28	—	—	1
TN	—	32	4	—
FP	—	1		—
FN	21	—	—	9
	I.S. 82/96		U.S. 65/96	
Accuracy	(85%)		(67%)	
Sensitivity	(83%)		(49%)	
Specificity	(89%)		(97%)	

36 antibody (1 mg) with imaging studies in a small number of patients with stage III/IV ovarian carcinoma. Scintigraphy was performed immediately following administration and before and after peritoneal lavage at 48 hours. Blood levels of both preparations were seen to rise over the first 20–40 hours, reaching 8–14% of the administered dose in the circulation, and then declined (T1/2 of 40 hours). Circulating radiolabel was still predominantly attached to antibody as shown by precipitation with anti-mouse IgG antiserum. There was little urinary excretion of In-111 (4% by 4 days) Figure 7.8. I-131 was excreted with T1/2 of 42 hours. Interpretation of the images was less clear than with previous studies using this antibody given i.v., but in some patients there was good agreement between the sites of uptake and the surgical findings. Measurement of the count rates from the images may be related to the whole body survival of the administered radioactivity by comparing Figures 7.8 and 7.9. The rapid appearance of ra-

TABLE 7.6C. Results of a European Multi-Centre Trial Comparing In-111-OC125 Immunoscintigraphy (I.S.) With C.T. and Ultrasound (C.T. and U.S.)

C.T. and U.S.	I.S.			
	TP	TN	FP	FN
TP	13	—	—	—
TN	—	16	3	—
FP	—	1		—
FN	11	—	—	5

	I.S. 41/49 (83%)	C.T. 39/66 32/49 (69%)
Accuracy		
Sensitivity	(82%)	(44%)
Specificity	(85%)	(95%)

diolabel in the bloodstream made it unclear as to whether tumour localisation was from circulating antibody rather than local infiltration. Tumour specimens resected at 4–5 days showed up to 0.05% of the dose/gram. These values may be plotted in histogram form to assess the uptake of radiolabels in resected tissues (Figure 7.10). This work and similar studies are now showing that the IP route of administration offers little advantage over the systemic route and may only be beneficial in the therapy of patients with ascites and malignant effusions. Overall, however, immunoscintigraphy should become a valuable clinical tool for the assessment of recurrent gynaecological cancer. This will ultimately depend upon the specificity of the monoclonal antibodies available.

Immunoscintigraphy of Breast Cancer

Carcinoma of the breast persists as one of the leading causes of cancer mortality in women living in the western world. Approximately 40% of all women with breast cancers develop overt recurrence or have died within 5 years of diagnosis. A number of parameters, such as tumour size, histological grade, presence of lymph node metastases, and serum marker status, are used to predict patient outcome. The antibody CA15.3, in particular, has been the most commonly used serum marker for the follow-up of patients with breast cancer. This antibody has not been demonstrated to be of any value for imaging, however. As with lung cancer, relatively few clinical studies have been undertaken to determine the use of immunoscintigraphy in the detection and monitoring of primary and metastatic breast cancer. Previous work on the immunoscintigraphy of breast cancer has been carried out with antibodies against CEA and HMFG. In 1982 De-

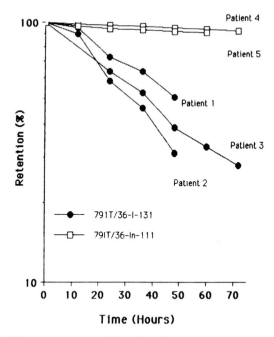

Fig. 7.8. Retention of radiolabelled 791T/36 antibody based on urinary excretion following intraperitoneal injection into 5 patients with recurrent ovarian carcinoma. (From the authors' unpublished studies.)

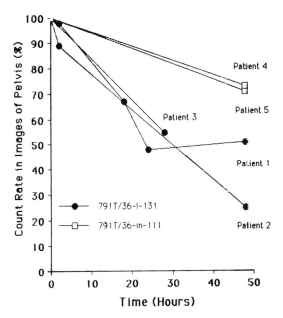

Fig. 7.9. Retention of radiolabelled antibody calculated from measured count rates in images of the same patients shown in Figure 7.8. (From the authors' unpublished studies.)

Land et al. detected 2 out of 5 primary mammary tumours and 7 out of 9 metastatic sites using I-131-labelled goat antibody to CEA. Epenetos et al. (1982) successfully imaged 4 out of 6 patients with extensive breast adenocarcinoma using I-123-labelled HMFG antibody. Ramsbury et al. (1983) used a similar antibody M8 labelled with In-111; however this study reported the visualisation of bone metastases rather than primary tumours. The authors carried out a pilot study in 1984 in 13 patients using the 791T/36 antibody labelled with I-131. This study demonstrated the deficiencies of the imaging technique with 3 out of 5 tumours visualised, and in one case a 9 cm diameter tumour was not detected. The use of emission tomography using In-111-791T/36 was subsequently found to improve tumour visualisation (Perkins et al., 1988). An example of

SPECT immunoscintigraphy of a primary breast tumour is given in Figure 7.11.

An additional approach for the *in vivo* use of antibodies is the detection of axillary lymph node involvement following subcutaneous injection of antibody. Tjandra et al. (1989) reported the use of I-131-labelled RCC-1 for the immunolymphoscintigraphy of lymph node metastases. This study involved the simultaneous administration of a second cold non-reactive antibody to block the uptake by normal nodes. This technique achieved a success rate of 86%, but it is unlikely to be used widely because of the co-administration of a second antibody.

The clinical use of immunoscintigraphy in the detection of primary breast cancer is extremely unlikely since mammography and ultrasound appear to have vastly superior resolution. The use of immunoscintigraphy in the detection of metastases and recurrent disease is still to be evaluated and may ultimately depend on the production of more specific antibodies. Of particular interest in this context is the work of Ryan et al. (1988) who used three human IgM monoclonal antibodies (YBM-209, YBY-088, and YBB-190) for the immunoscintigraphy of metastatic breast carcinoma. This study is of interest since it is considered to be the first reported use of In-111-human IgM monoclonal antibody for imaging metastatic disease. Sites of metastatic disease were accurately identified in patients in whom YBM-209 or YBY-088 was used.

Immunoscintigraphy of Lung Cancer

Carcinoma of the lung is one of the major cancer types, and statistics show that the incidence of this disease is increasing. Following initial diagnosis the 5-year survival for patients is less than 10%. Carcinoma of

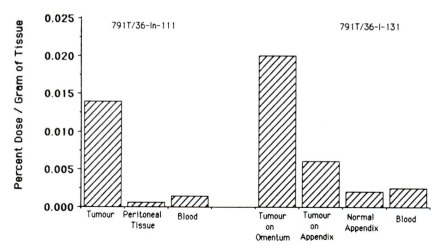

Fig. 7.10. Percent injected dose per gram of tissue in two patients with recurrent ovarian carcinoma following intraperitoneal injection of In-111- or I-131-791T/36 antibody. (From the authors' unpublished studies.)

the bronchus falls into one of four main histological types: squamous cell (epidermoid), large cell (non-differential), adenocarcinoma, and small cell (anaplastic). The major form of therapy for squamous cell carcinoma and adenocarcinoma is surgery, whereas radiation therapy and chemotherapy are applied in the remainder of cases.

A large number of antibodies reactive with bronchial carcinoma have been produced (see Appendix: Antibody Look-Up Table, this volume) and much *in vitro*

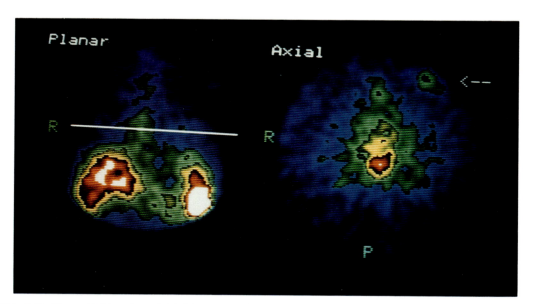

Fig. 7.11. Planer (left) and axial (right) images of a patient with a 5 cm primary tumour of the left breast recorded 48 hours following injection of 1 mg (80 MBq/2 mCi) In-111-791T/36 antibody. Activity can be seen in the liver, spleen, spine, sternum, and tumour (arrow). The horizontal line shows the position of the axial cut.

work carried out. However, comparatively little work has been published on the immunoscintigraphy of primary lung carcinoma. Goldenberg and DeLand (1982) reviewed positive results in 18 out of 25 patients with primary lung cancer using I-131-labelled polyclonal anti-CEA antibodies, whereas polyclonal antibody raised against alpha-fetoprotein failed to detect lung carcinoma in three patients. Further analysis of the detection of lung tumours by DeLand (1982) showed that variation in the level of detection was more related to the size and location of the lesion rather than tumour histology. In their study antibody imaging detected over 90% of lesions greater than 2 cm in diameter but only 40% of lesions less than this size, and the histology of the tumour showed no correlation with the accuracy of detection. In 1986 the authors published imaging studies in a small number of patients with primary small cell and squamous cell lung tumours using the 791T/36 antibody. The main conclusion from his study was that the detection of lung tumours varied depending on the radiolabel and imaging technique employed. Three out of 8 patients imaged with I-131 antibody showed positive findings, whereas 9 out of 13 patients imaged with In-111-labelled antibody were positive. Emission tomography increased the detection rate even further. However, the results from all these published studies indicate that it is unlikely that anti-CEA, AFP, or 791T/36 antibodies are capable of offering clinically useful information to patients with primary lung cancer.

More promising studies have employed monoclonal antibodies raised directly against lung tumours, although some results have been disappointing. For example, Mathieu et al. (1984) raised a monoclonal antibody directly against squamous cell lung cancer, which showed high in vi-

tro reactivity to lung tumour cells and weak cross-reactivity with normal lung tissues. However, imaging using I-131 as the radiolabel failed to show localisation by either planar or single photon emission tomography. A number of different methods have been used in order to produce antibodies with greater specificity for lung tumours. Some studies have involved the immortalisation of B lymphocytes taken from patients with lung cancer using Epstein-Barr virus or fusion with a plasmocytoma and have resulted in human monoclonal antibodies of the IgM class. Reviewing other published reports, over 20 murine monoclonal antibodies raised against either small cell or squamous cell lung cancer have been raised and the antibodies SWA11 and Po66, in particular, would appear important candidate antibodies for immunoscintigraphy. Preliminary results for I-131-Po66 in 33 patients with non-small cell lung cancer showed a detection rate of 78% for primary tumours and 100% for recurrences (Bourguet et al., 1990).

Overall, imaging studies in this type of cancer have not been as encouraging as those in the other major cancer types—for example, colorectal and ovarian tumours. Imaging studies for the detection of lung metastases from other sites would appear to be of greater value. Work is currently underway to develop a serum marker based on one of these antibodies which would be more specific or lung cancer. At the present time, therefore, the role of immunoscintigraphy in the detection of lung cancer remains to be determined.

Immunoscintigraphy of Melanoma

Malignant melanoma is an extremely aggressive cancer. Patients with disseminated disease seldom live for longer than 12 months following diagnosis. The early detection of small lesions is therefore crucial if patient survival is to be improved. A large number of melanoma-associated antigens (MAA) have been described, some reacting with cytoplasmic components of the melanoma cells and others reacting with plasma membranes. The antigens which have received the most attention for immunoscintigraphy are the p97 antigen and the high-molecular-weight melanoma-associated antigens (HMW-MAA). The p97 antigen (97,000 molecular weight cell surface glycoprotein) has been rigorously characterised, and over 13 antibodies which react with 5 different p97 epitopes have been generated.

Two antibodies raised against HMW-MAA, 9.2.27 and 225.28S, have been used extensively. Antibody 225.28S is directed against a plasma membrane glycoprotein antigen of molecular weights 280kDa and 440kDa and appears a most suitable antibody for imaging purposes. Much work was carried out on this antibody during the 1980s by the Italian groups with the support of Sorin Biomedica (Salaggia, Italy), and a range of I-123, In-111, and Tc-99m intact antibodies, F(ab')$_2$ and Fab fragments were investigated clinically. Out of an extremely large number of studies, F(ab')$_2$ fragments radiolabelled with Tc-99m or In-111 emerged as the most appropriate immunoradiopharmaceuticals for the detection of metastatic melanoma. A report comprising studies in over 200 patients using the antibody 225.28S (Siccardi et al., 1986) concluded that the immunoscintigraphy of melanoma was a reliable procedure, detecting over 70% of lesions. Since more than half of the metastatic deposits from primary melanoma are situated in the skin and superficial lymph nodes immunoscintigraphy would appear an attractive proposition, however, the detection of small lesions less than 5 mm remains difficult, especially if the sites of disease are situated centrally in the body, or even in the main trunk. Nonspecific uptake

in bone marrow, liver, spleen, and kidneys remains a problem, since this may mask the uptake of antibody in tumour sites. The detection of ocular melanoma would appear to be a particularly promising application for immunoscintigraphy. Published studies (Bomangi et al., 1987; Scheidhauer et al., 1988) have demonstrated the accurate detection of tumours down to as small as 2 mm in diameter. Detection rates of over 70% may be achieved if emission tomography is performed. Figure 7.12 shows an example of the immunoscintigraphy of ocular melanoma using Tc-99m-225.28S F(ab')$_2$ fragments. If used in combination with other diagnostic tests, it is thought that immunoscintigraphy may be capable of differentiating uveal melanoma from other similar tumours of the eye.

Immunoscintigraphy of Other Malignancies

Monoclonal antibodies have been raised and used for the detection of a number of malignancies other than the major cancer types mentioned above. The number of antibodies available continues to grow. The other main applications include the detection of thyroid tumours, bone and soft tissue tumours, neural tumours, and the detection and treatment of cerebrospinal tumours.

The immunoscintigraphy of medullary thyroid cancer has been attempted with anti-CEA antibodies and antibodies reacting against calcitonin such as CTO3, CTO6, and KCO1. At the time of writing this work is at a preliminary stage and patient numbers are limited. Further clinical studies are necessary to determine whether these antibodies will replace the more conventional diagnostic agents.

Acute lymphoblastic leukaemia and primary brain tumours are relatively common tumours of children. Antibodies such as UJ13A and UJ181.4 raised against foetal brain tissue have been investigated for the detection of tumours of the brain and CSF pathway (Richardson et al., 1986). These antibodies do not appear to be of value in the detection and staging of these tumours but have been used in preliminary studies for guided radiotherapy after intrathecal injection. Immunoscintigraphy also appears capable of imaging metastatic neuroblastoma. Studies have been carried out by Baum et al., 1989, using BW595/9 antibody. This antibody was originally raised against small cell lung cancer cells but was shown to react immunohistochemically with a high percentage of neuroblastomas. An example showing the use of Tc-99m-BW595/9 antibody in comparison with MIBG is given in Figure 7.13. A wide range of other tumour types have been investigated with variable results. In some cases the tumours are relatively rare and, as a result, have not received much attention. This is sometimes due to the low numbers of patients available for clinical evaluation of the antibody.

In the liver immunoscintigraphy has mainly been applied for the detection of liver metastases. Demangeat et al. (1988) investigated 41 patients with primary hepatoma using I-123 anti-alpha-fetoprotein. Low detection rates were achieved with a sensitivity of 53% and a specificity of 67%. The detection and staging of other tumour types may ultimately prove to be of clinical value, an example being the detection of Hodgkin's Disease using a Hodgkin-associated monoclonal antibody HRS-1 (Carde et al., 1990). Further information on the application of monoclonal antibodies in other pathologies may be obtained from the Appendix: Antibody Look-Up Table, this volume.

IMMUNOSCINTIGRAPHY IN BENIGN DISEASE
Cardiovascular Disease

Myocardial infarction. The first monoclonal antibody preparation for the imaging of benign disease was raised against intracellular myosin and is secreted by hybridoma R11D10. Myoscint (mifarmonab, Centocor Inc.) is a monoclonal antibody Fab fragment coupled with DTPA for radiolabelling with In-111-indium chloride. This antibody binds specifically to intracellular myosin which becomes exposed as a result of cell death. Following intravenous injection, this antibody proves capable of assessing the extent and severity of myocardial necrosis and has been shown to be more accurate than pyrophosphate for the delineation of infarct size. A review of the application of antimyosin antibodies has been made by Johnson and Sedin (1989).

Clinical studies have shown the total plasma clearance of myoscint to be biphasic with an initial half-time of 2 hours and a subsequent half-time of 26 hours. Being a monovalent fragment, the major route of clearance from the body is via the kidneys, these being the critical organs which receive the order of 0.3 mGy/MBq (14.5 Rad/mCi). Few minor reactions have been reported following intravenous administration, these being fever, chest pain, headache, nausea, and vomiting. No cases of HAMA have been reported in the sera of patients receiving this antibody preparation. Imaging is normally performed 18–24 hours following injection of 80 MBq (2 mCi). Three sets of planar views are usually recorded in the anterior 45°, left anterior oblique, and left lateral projections. The overall sensitivity for patients with transmural myocardial infarction is 91%, which reduces to 76% in patients with non-transmural myocardial infarction. Specificities of over 90% have been achieved, with an overall diagnostic accuracy of around 90%. One of the main limitations of antimyosin is the absence of any information concerning the normal myocardium. This can lead to difficulty for the accurate assessment of the site of lesions.

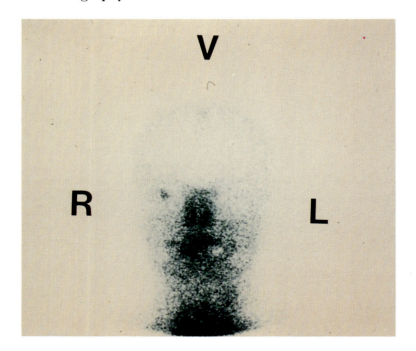

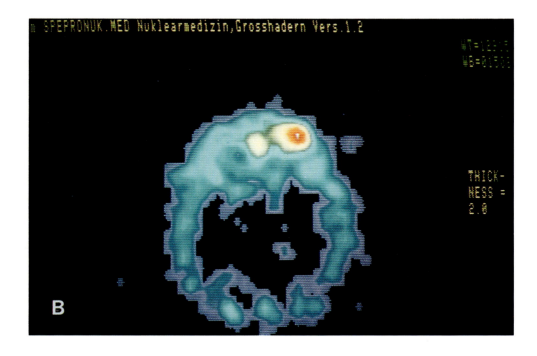

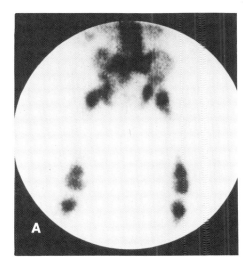 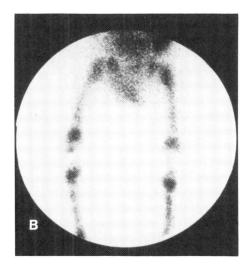

Fig. 7.13. **A:** I-123 Meta-iodo-benzylguanidine images of the pelvis and lower extremities of a 2-year-old child with metastatic neuroblastoma (Stage IV) recorded six hours post injection. Diffuse bone marrow metastases can be seen. **B:** Immunoscintigraphy using Tc-99m-labelled BW575/9 antibody in the same patient recorded 7 hours after administration. This study was performed 3 months after the images shown in A and after several courses of chemotherapy. Intense uptake can be seen in multiple bone marrow metastases confirming chemotherapy resistant cells (proven by biopsy). (Study provided by Dr. R.P. Baum, Assistant Professor of Nuclear Medicine, University Hospital, Frankfurt, FRG.)

Dual radionuclide imaging using Tl-201 and antimyosin has been advocated in some instances for complete assessment of the myocardium. It is thought that this may be especially useful following myocardial infarction or thrombolytic therapy.

Abnormal antimyosin studies have been found in patients with unstable angina, acute myocarditis, chronic dilated cardiomyopathy, and cardiac transplant rejection. The uptake pattern is usually quite different from the normal in such cases, being diffuse in nature. A heart-to-lung uptake ratio has been used for quantification, with a value of the order of 1.5 in normal subjects. Ratios of between 1.6 and 5 have

been found in patients with myocyte necrosis. It is also interesting to note that antimyosin has been used for the immunoscintigraphy of rhabdomyosarcoma, although the clinical utility of this application remains to be proven.

Transplant rejection. The diagnosis of acute rejection after cardiac transplantation is considered to be a clinically useful application for antimyosin antibody. The absence of HAMA following the clinical administration of this antibody fragment indicates that repeat studies may be undertaken, safely reducing the need for endomyocardial biopsy. The use of this and other antibodies for the early assess-

Fig. 7.12. Immunoscintigraphy of ocular melanoma. **A:** Planar. **B:** SPECT images demonstrating the use of Tc-99m F(ab')$_2$ fragments of the anti-melanoma antibody 225-285 in patients with ocular melanoma. Patients were injected with 250 μg antibody radiolabelled with 800 MBq (22 mCi) Tc-99m and imaged within 22 hours of injection. (Images supplied by Dr. K. Scheidhauer, University of Munster Klinik and Politechnik, Munster, FRG.)

ment of organ rejection offers new horizons for the management of patients undergoing organ transplantation. Anti-T-cell antibodies represent a group of antibodies with an important clinical role in this context. The anti-T-cell antibody produced by Behringwerke, FRG (BW111, IgG1) is directed against a 50 kDa epitope on human T-cells (pan T-ERCF receptor present on 80% of all peripheral blood lymphocytes). Following injection of 0.1–1 mg of intact Tc-99m-labelled BW111 antibody into 7 kidney transplant patients Hertel et al. (1990) reported intense uptake in all patients with acute cell-mediated kidney rejection. Normal kidneys showed no abnormal uptake. This study opens up a promising new area of application for antibody imaging.

Thrombus detection. A variety of investigations exists for the detection of thromboembolic disease, including X-ray arteriography, radionuclide angiography, and pulmonary imaging and Doppler ultrasound. In patients with a suspicion of thromboembolism it is desirable to assess three main parameters: Site, extent, and maturity (i.e., whether the lesion is active or chronic). A number of radiopharmaceuticals have previously been used for the detection of thrombosis and thromboembolism. These materials have been associated with different stages of thrombogenesis, such as radiolabelled platelets for imaging haemostasis, radiolabelled fibrin or fibrinogen for the detection of coagulation, and radiolabelled streptokinase and heparin for the detection of fibrinolysis. Monoclonal antibodies have been generated with high *in vivo* specificity for platelets, activated platelet factor, and fibrin (see Table 7.7). A review of the status of

TABLE 7.7. Antibodies Used for Imaging Thrombus and Thromboembolism Categorised by Target Antigen

Platelet-specific antibodies		
Target Antigen	Antibody	Reference
IIb/IIIa receptor	P256	Bai et al. (1984)
	7E3	Coller et al. (1983)
	10E3	Coller et al. (1983)
	50H.19	Som et al. (1986)
Activated platelet factor	Anti-GMP140	McEver et al. (1984)
	S12	McEver et al. (1984)
	anti-TSP/TSP1.1	Legrand et al. (1988)
Fibrin-specific antibodies		
Amino terminus of fibrin II	64C5	Hui et al. (1985)
	59D8	Hui et al. (1983)
	T2G1s	Kudryk et al. (1984)
	anti-fbn-17	Scheefers-Borchel et al. (1985)
	DD-3B6-22	Rylatt et al. (1983)

From Koblik et al., 1989.

these materials has been made by Koblik et al. (1989).

Platelet-specific antibodies. These have been successfully used for the immunoscintigraphy of thrombus and thromboembolism. These have primarily been directed against a 135,000 molecular weight glycoprotein IIb/IIIa membrane receptor complex which is thought to function in platelet aggregation and serves as a receptor for fibrinogen. The GPIIb/IIIa complex is one of many similar glycoprotein receptors that mediate adhesion phenomena in a wide range of cell types, such as endothelial cells, granulocytes, monocytes, and fibroblasts. Antibodies such as 7E3, 50H.19, P256, and B59.2 appear to offer potential for imaging (Koblik et al., 1989). *In vitro* and experimental studies show that this group of antibodies will bind to resting platelets but that the IIb/IIIa epitope is expressed to a greater extent on activated platelets. Some cross-reaction with monocytes has also been reported (Bai et al., 1984), although the P256 antibody appears to react with platelets only. There is evidence that some of these antibodies will affect platelet aggregation and adhesion. Experiments using large doses of antibody 7E3 antibody (0.2 mg/Kg) have shown a blocking effect on platelet aggregation, and this anti-thrombotic effect has been used to accelerate cardiac thrombolysis. The P256 antibody when used in the intact form (IgG1) has been shown to cause platelet aggregation *in vitro* (Stuttle et al., 1988). The bivalent $F(ab')_2$ fragment also showed some aggregation of platelets; however, the Fab' fragment caused no platelet aggregation and is therefore considered appropriate for clinical use.

Indium-111- and I-123-labelled antibodies directed against the IIb/IIIa glycoprotein complex have been shown to have similar blood clearance kinetics, with 50% of the dose being cleared one hour following intravenous injection. As would be expected, urinary clearance of iodine-labelled antibody is greater than that of indium-labelled antibody. The blood clearance of Tc-99m-Fab' and $F(ab')_2$ fragments have been reported to be far greater with 50% clearance in less than 6 minutes. Clot to blood ratios as high as 120:1 have been reported from post mortem investigations (Oster et al., 1985; Thakur, 1988). Imaging studies have demonstrated that clots may be visualised from 15 minutes post-injection, although some studies have been carried out up to 48 hours using In-111-labelled antibodies. The P256 antibody has probably been used more extensively for clinical imaging and has been shown to be of clinical value in the detection of venous thrombosis (Peters et al., 1986; Stuttle et al., 1988), pulmonary embolism (Stuttle et al., 1989), and arterial thrombus (Perkins et al., 1990). Typically 100 μg In-111-Fab' fragments (20MBq) have been used and images have been obtained at between 3 and 24 hours. An example of the use of In-111-P256Fab' in peripheral arterial thrombi is given in Figure 7.14. In addition to localisation of thrombi, the use of this antibody appears to offer information on the maturity of the thrombi, with the clots of more recent origin showing uptake more rapidly following injection. Published studies have shown that imaging with P256 antibody is positive for active thrombi, whereas the older more chronic thrombi (generally of greater than 30 days duration) are not detected. Hence, it would appear that immunoscintigraphy using platelet-specific antibody can offer additional information to arteriography. This information is especially valuable in patients presenting with arterial thromboses, where the new clot busting agents such as streptokinase and tissue plasminogen activator (tPA) appear to be of value for thrombolysis. The use of these antibodies would

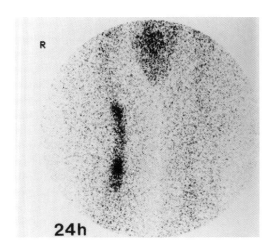

24h

Fig. 7.14. Anterior view of the thighs of a 59-year-old male with a long history of peripheral vascular disease who presented with a 3-day history of a cold right leg. Image recorded 24 hours following injection of 100 μg P256 Fab' platelet specific antibody radiolabelled with 20 MBq (0.5 mCi) In-111. Marked uptake is visible along the mid portion of the right superficial femoral artery.

therefore appear to offer a means of selecting patients presenting with peripheral arterial thrombosis who are suitable for thrombolytic therapy and would therefore be a valuable investigation in patients presenting with arterial occlusion.

Antibodies against activated platelet factors (GMP140, S12 and anti-TSP) appear to perform in a similar manner to those directed against the GP IIb/IIIa receptor. Antibodies raised against alpha granule membrane protein (GMP), which is expressed on platelet plasma membrane during activation-dependent granulation, have been used experimentally for the detection of sites of vascular injury (McEver et al., 1984; Palabrica et al., 1989).

Antibodies reacting with thrombospondin (TSP) have also been examined in experimental models. TSP is a 400 kDa protein which is secreted in alpha granules by activated platelets. This acts as a glue for platelet aggregation. TSP binds in small

amounts to resting platelets but is increased up to sevenfold in activated platelets. The optimum imaging time with these agents is considered to be of the order of 6 hours.

Further studies are required to evaluate the relative performance and clinical potential of this group of antibodies. To date, it would appear that regardless of the mechanism involved, antibodies reacting with platelets are more useful during the acute phase of thrombogenesis when platelet aggregation is taking place.

Fibrin-specific antibodies. These have been found to generally react against the amino terminal of the B chain of fibrin II. The first reports on the production of antibodies directed against fibrin and fibrinogen were published in the early 1980s. Murine antibodies against fibrinogen have been produced from mice immunised with a surprising range of materials—for example, monoblastic leukaemia cells, Factor VIII complex, and the urine from patients with bladder cancer. Many of these antibodies have subsequently been used as biological probes for the determination of the structure of the fibrinogen molecule. The antibodies which have been shown to offer the greatest clinical potential are mainly IgG1 antibodies reacting with fibrin: T2G1s, 59D8, 64C5, and Y22. Once injected, the clearance rates of these antibodies either as intact IgG or F(ab')$_2$ and radiolabelled with In-111 or I-131 are similar, with clearance half-times of 25–30 hours, resulting in high background activity seen on images. Fab fragments have a half-time clearance of the order of 15 hours. The absence of any cross-reaction of these antibodies with circulating fibrinogen makes them ideal for clot imaging. Early anti-fibrin imaging carried out in animal models shows intense hepatic uptake, which is considered to be due to nonspecific Fc receptors in the reticuloendothelial cells. Images of In-111 and Tc-99m labelled fragments also show high early-phase renal activity. Most intravascular experimental clots have been visualised by 48 hours following administration. The T2G1s and 59D8 antibodies have received the most clinical attention and appear to perform best as Tc-99m-Fab′ fragments. Typically, 0.5 mg Fab′ fragments radiolabelled with 550–750 MBq (15–20 mCi) Tc-99m. Sensitivities of 100% have been reported for the detection of deep vein thrombosis.

From the information currently available, both platelet-specific and anti-fibrin antibodies are capable of imaging sites of thrombus formation. Arterial thrombi tend to be rich in platelets and low in fibrin. It is expected, therefore, that anti-platelet antibodies should be more suitable for the detection of arterial thromboses. Thrombi forming in veins with slower moving blood contain more fibrin and should be visualised more effectively with anti-fibrin antibodies. Anti-fibrin is also considered to more suitable for the detection of clots irrespective of their age. Experimental studies in a canine model has demonstrated the superiority of platelet antibody over that of fibrin antibody (Palabricia et al., 1989), and clot-to-blood ratios are generally higher with platelet specific antibody. It would appear that the clinical use of these antibodies also provides information on the stage of the thrombus, although uptake is variable, depending on treatment that has been initiated at the time of the investigation. For example, intravenous heparin is considered to reduce the uptake of platelet-specific antibodies, whereas some of the fibrin epitopes are unaffected by anticoagulant therapy. Clearly, the clinical use of these agents is likely to expand dramatically during the near future.

Infection and Inflammation

The detection of sites of tissue inflammation within the body often presents a difficult diagnostic problem. If the process has reached an advanced stage, imaging techniques such as ultrasound and X-ray CT are of great importance to the physician. Patients who persist with pyrexia of unknown origin present a difficult diagnostic problem, and radionuclide imaging can be especially helpful in these cases. Gallium-67 citrate was for many years the conventional agent for imaging sites of inflammatory disease. The sensitivity and specificity of this radiopharmaceutical varies widely (50–100%). In recent years the use of radiolabelled leucocytes has been advocated, initially using In-111-indium oxine and more recently using Tc-99m-HMPAO, although these radiolabelling procedures require time-consuming manipulations within the radiopharmacy, such as differential centrifugation, incubation, washing, and resuspension.

The aim of the immunoscintigraphy of inflammation is ultimately the targeting of antibodies directed against microbial specific antigens. However, antibodies that have been used previously for the clinical detection of inflammation and abscess have been largely non-specific. The binding of some anti-CEA antibodies with the non-specific cross-reacting antigen, NCA-95, which is expressed on the majority of granulocytes, has led to the use of these agents for the detection of abscess and inflammation. The antibody CEA-A47 initially raised by Mach in Switzerland has since been developed into a lyophilised kit for radiolabelling with Tc-99m (BI71.015 Granuloscint, Hoechst, Wiesbaden, Federal Republic of Germany). Approximately 26% of the radioactivity spontaneously binds to granulocytes in the circulation and 14% remains in the plasma (Locher et al., 1986). However, up to 60% of the activity accumulates in the bone marrow, which is a feature of other anti-granulocyte antibodies. A similar preparation radiolabelled with I-123 is also available in Europe through the Mallinkrodt Company. The other main antibody which has been used for *in vivo* radiolabelling of granulocytes is the BW 250/183, which also cross reacts with NCA-95. This antibody produced by Behringwerke (Marburg, Federal Republic of Germany) has been used extensively in patients using Tc-99m as the radiolabel, for the detection of abscess and inflammation. This antibody has been shown to bind to about 95% of human granulocytes, although measurements on blood samples taken 6 hours following administration have shown only around 25% of the radioactivity bound to granulocytes (Joseph et al., 1988). *In vitro* studies have shown that the BW 250/183 antibody does not affect the normal physiological function of the granulocytes, which is in contrast to other NCA-binding antibodies such as BW 241/10, which have a strong inhibitory affect on normal as well as stimulated granulocytes. Published studies show that the BW 250/183 antibody has a similar specificity and sensitivity to radiolabelled leucocytes for the detection of abscess and inflammation. Studies have been carried out in patients with bone infection, inflammatory bowel disease, pancreatitis, and bone marrow lesions. However, this antibody is unable to differentiate between septic and non-septic inflammation. Although the BW 250/183 is radiolabelled with Tc-99m, unlike Tc-99m-HMPAO-labelled leucocytes, there is no excretion through the biliary tract, and therefore images recorded at 24 hours after injection are commonly per-

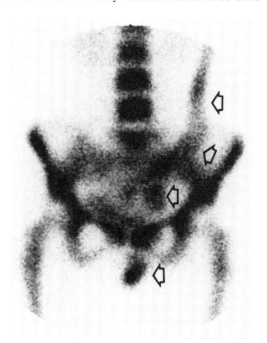

Fig. 7.15. Anterior view of the pelvis and lower abdomen of a 31-year-old female patient with Crohns disease. Image recorded 6 hours following administration of 200 MBq (5.4 mCi) Tc-99m-BW250/183 (Granulozyt) antibody. Increased uptake can be seen in the descending and sigmoid colon and rectum. Uptake can also be seen in a peri-anal abscess (**lower arrow**). (High uptake in bone marrow is a normal feature of these studies).

TABLE 7.8. Monoclonal Antibodies Specific for Human Neutrophils

Antibody	Isotype
B.37.2.1	IgM
MCA 161	IgG1
FMC 11	IgG1
FMC 14	IgM
MCA 87	IgG2a
MCA 149 A	IgG1
MCA 215	IgM
MCA 167	IgG2a
anti-SSEA-1	IgM
B.6.2	IgG

From Thakur et al., 1988.

formed and have been found particularly helpful. Typically, doses of 1 mg of antibody radiolabelled with 300 MBq (8 mCi) Tc-99m are given. An example of a patient with inflammatory bowel disease is shown in Figure 7.15. Further characteristics of this antibody preparation are the relatively low uptake in normal liver but high uptake in bone when compared with In-111 and Tc-99m-HMPAO-labelled leucocytes. This has enabled the detection of liver abscesses and the use of the antibody for bone marrow imaging.

There remains a need for antibodies directed to sub-populations of cells in order to increase diagnostic specificity. A num-

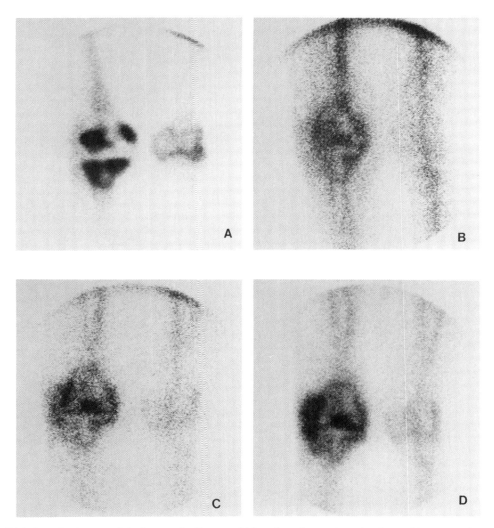

Fig. 7.16. Anterior images of the knees of a 70-year-old female with an infected right total knee prosthesis. A: Tc-99m-MDP bone image 4 hours after injection. B, C, D: 4 hours (B), 24 hours (C), and 48 hours (D) following injection of 1 mg, 75 MBq (2 mCi) In-111-DTPA polyclonal immunoglobulin G (Sandoglobulin). (Study provided by Dr. W.I.G. Ogen and Professor F.H.M. Corstens, Sint Rudboudziekenhuis, University of Nigmegen, Netherlands.)

ber of antibodies have been raised against
neutrophils, and attempts to develop them
as radiopharmaceuticals have been reported by Thakur et al., 1988. Of ten antibodies investigated (Table 7.8), one
antibody raised against stage specific em-
bryonic antigen (SSEA-1) appeared the
most promising as a radiolabelled preparation for *in vivo* use.

**Human non-specific gamma globu-
lin (HIG).** It is commonly perceived that

one of the major limitations of murine
monoclonal antibodies for the diagnosis of
benign conditions such as abscess and inflammation is the possibility of human
anti-mouse antibody (HAMA). Recently
In-111-1 and Tc-99m-labelled human non-
specific polyclonal immunoglobulin (HIG)
have been used for the detection of focal
infections (Oyen et al., 1989; Buscombe et
al., 1990). One particular preparation,
Sandoglobulin, has been licensed in the

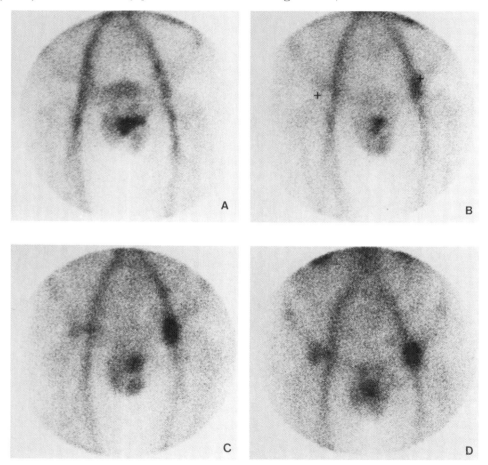

Fig. 7.17. Anterior images of a 65-year-old patient with an infected aorta-bifemoral bypass graft following
injection of 1 mg 75 MBq (2 mCi) In-111-DTPA-polyclonal immunoglobulin G (Sandoglobulin). **A:** 4 hours. **B:**
24 hours. **C:** 48 hours following injection. **D:** 72 hours following injection. Increasing uptake is seen in both
distal anastomoses of the bypass, but this is more prominent on the left side. The markers in the 24 hour image
show the sites of the fistulae. (Images provided by Dr. W.J.G. Oyen and Professor F.H.M. Corstens, Sint
Rudboudziekenhuis, University of Nigmegen, Netherlands.)

United States by the Food and Drug administration for the purpose of treating immune-deficient conditions. One of the main advantage of imaging with this type of material is that they are of human origin and will not therefore result in the production of HAMA. The non-specific binding of these materials is thought to be via the Fc portion of the immunoglobulin. Typically 75 MBq (2 mCi) In-111-DTPA-HIG or 200 MBq (5 mCi) Tc-99m-HIG is administered. At 1 hour following injection, the blood pool activity is high. By 4 hours the blood pool activity of both radiolabelled preparations is decreased with liver, spleen, kidneys, and bladder remaining as areas of highest uptake. Immunoscintigraphy using polyclonal HIG has demonstrated positive identification of inflammation in a variety of conditions and is thought to be of particular value in the assessment of patients with febrile neutropenia. However, discrimination between infection and sterile inflammatory lesions does not appear possible (Oyen et al., 1989). Two example of the use of In-111-HIG are given in Figures 7.16 and 7.17.

REFERENCES AND FURTHER READING

Abdel-Nabi, H.H., Ortam-Nabi, J.A., See, W., Lee, J., Ireton, R., Boileau, M., Unger, M.W., Halverson, C. (1990): Clinical experience with intra lymphatic administration of ^{111}In-labelled monoclonal antibody PAY 276 for the detection of pelvic nodal metastases in prostatic carcinoma. Eur. J. Nucl. Med. 16:149–156.

Abdel-Nabi, H.H., Schwartz, A.N., Higano, C.S., Wechter, D.G., Unger, M.W. (1987): Colorectal carcinoma: Detection with indium-111 anticarcinoembryonic-antigen monoclonal antibody ZCE-025. Radiology 164:617–621.

Armitage, N.C., Perkins, A.C., Durrant, L.G., Ellis, I.O., Ballantyne, K.C., Harrison, R.C., Riley, A.M.L., Robins, R.A., Wastie, M.L., Hardcastle, J.D. (1986): The in vitro binding and in vivo localisation in colorectal cancer of a high affinity monoclonal antibody to carcinoembryonic antigen. Br. J. Surg. 73:965–969.

Armitage, N.C., Perkins, A.C., Pimm, M.V., Farrands, P.A., Baldwin, R.W., Hardcastle, J.D. (1984): The localisation of an anti-tumour monoclonal antibody (791T/36) in gastrointestinal tumours. Br. J. Surg. 71:407–412.

Armitage, N.C., Perkins, A.C., Pimm, M.V., Wastie, M.L., Baldwin, R.W., Hardcastle, J.D. (1985): Imaging of primary and metastatic colorectal cancer using an In-111-labelled anti-tumour monoclonal antibody 791T/36. Nucl. Med. Commun. 6:623–631.

Bai, Y., Durbin, H., Hogg, N. (1984): Monoclonal antibodies specific for platelet glycoproteins react with human monocytes. Blood 64:139–146.

Barzen, G., Mayr, A.C., Langer, M., Becker, R., Cordes, M., Zwicker, C., Koppenhagen, K., Felix, R. (1989): Radioimmunoscintigraphy of ovarian cancer with 131-iodine labelled OC-125 antibody fragments. Eur. J. Nucl. Med. 15:42–48.

Baum, R.P., Hertel, A., Lorenz, M., Schwarz, A., Encke, A., Har, G. (1989): Tc-99m-labelled anti-CEA monoclonal antibody for tumour immunoscintigraphy: First clinical results. Nucl. Med. Commun. 5:345–352.

Begent, R.H.J., Keep, P., Searle, F., Green, A.J., Mitchell, H.D.C., Jones, B.E., Dent, J., Pendower, J.E.H., Parkins, R.A., Reynolds, K.W.Q., Cooke, T.G., Mersh, T.A., Bagshawe, K.D. (1986): Radioimmunolocalization and selection for surgery in recurrent colorectal cancer. Br. J. Surg. 73:64–67.

Bomangi, J., Hungerford, J.L., Granowska, M., Britton, K.E. (1987): Radioimmunoscintigraphy of ocular melanoma with Tc-99m labelled cutaneous melanoma antibody fragments. Br. J. Ophthalmol. 71:651–658.

Bosslet, K., Luben, G., Schwarz, A., Hundt, E., Harthus, H.P., Seiler, F.R., Muhrer, C., Kloppel, G., Kayser, K., Sedlacek, H.H. (1985): Immunohistochemical localization and molecular characteristics of three monoclonal antibody-defined epitopes detectable on carcinoembryonic antigen (CEA). Int. J. Cancer. 36:75–84.

Bourguet, P., Dazord, L., Desrues, B., Collet, B., Ramee, M.P., Delaval, P., Martin, A., Logeais, Y., Pelletier, A., Toujas, L., Bourel, D., Kernec, J., Saccavini, J.C., Kremer, M., Herr, J.Y. (1990): Immunoscintigraphy of human lung squamous cell carcinoma using an iodine-131 labelled monoclonal antibody (Po66). Br. J. Cancer 61:230–234.

Buraggi, G.L., Crippa, F., Gasparini, M., Seregni, E., Presti, M., Marini, A., Fontanelli, R.V., Colnaghi, M.I. (1989): Preliminary results of the first diagnostic applications of a monoclonal antibody against ovarian cancer (MOV 18): Eur. J. Nucl. Med. 15:C1 (Abstract).

Buscombe, J.R., Lui, D., Ensing, G., de Jong, R., Ell, P.J. (1990): Tc-99m-human immunoglobulin (HIG)—first results of a new agent for the localization of infection and inflammation. Eur. J. Nucl. Med. 16:649–655.

Carde, P., Da Costa, L., Manil, L., Pfreundschuh, M., Lumbroso, J.D., Saccavini, J.C., Caillou, B., Ricard, M., Boudet, F., Hayat, M., Diehl, V., Parmentier, C. (1990): Immunoscintigraphy of Hodgkins Disease: *In-vivo* use of radiolabelled monoclonal antibodies derived from Hodgkins cell lines. Eur. J. Cancer 26:474–479.

Chatal, J-F., Saccavini, J.C., Fumoleau, P., Douillard, Y-Y., Curtet, C., Kremer, M., Le Mevel, B., Kaproski, H. (1984): Immunoscintigraphy of colon carcinoma. J. Nucl. Med. 25:307–314.

Colcher, D., Esteban, J.M., Carrasquillo, J.A., Sugarbaker, P., Reynolds, J.C., Bryant, G., Larson, S.M., Schlom, J. (1987): Quantitative analysis of selective radiolabelled monoclonal antibody localisation in metastatic lesions of colorectal cancer patients. Cancer Res. 47:1185.

Coller, B.S., Folts, J.D., Smith, S.R., Scudder, L.E., Jordan, R. (1989): Abolition of in vivo platelet thrombus formation in primates with monoclonal antibodies to the platelet GPIIb/IIIa receptor. Correlation with bleeding time, platelet aggregation and blockage of GPIIb/IIIa receptors. Circulation 80:1766–1774.

Coller, B.S., Peerschke, E.I., Scudder, L.E., Sullivan, C.A. (1983): A murine monoclonal antibody that completely blocks the binding of fibrinogen to platelets produces a thrombasthenic-like state in normal platelets and bind to glycoproteins IIb and/or IIIa. J. Clin. Invest. 72:325–338.

Davies, J.O., Davies, E.R., Howe, K., Jackson, P.C., Pitcher, E.M., Sadowski, C.S., Stirrat, G.M., Sunderland, C.A. (1985): Radionuclide imaging of ovarian tumours with 123I-labelled monoclonal antibody (ND0G2) directed against placental alkaline phosphate. Br. J. Obstet. Gynaecol. 92:277–286.

Delaloye, B., Bischof-Delaloye, A., Buchegger, F., von Fleidner, V., Grob, J-F., Volant, J-C., Pettavel, J., Mach, J-P. (1986): Detection of colorectal carcinoma by emission-computerized tomography after injection of I-123-labelled Fab or (Fab')₂ fragments from monoclonal anti carcinoembryonic antigen antibodies. J. Clin. Invest. 77:301–311.

DeLand, F.H., Kim, E.E., Goldenberg, D.H. (1982): *In vivo* radioimmunodetection of cancer. In: Wilson, C.G., Hardy, J.G., Frier, M., Davis, S.S. (eds.): London: Croom Helm, pp. 181–202. Radionuclide Imaging in Drug Research.

Demangeat, J.L., Manil, L., Demangeat, C., Rico, E., Stadel-Flaig, C., Duclos, B., Brunot, B., Jaeck, D., Bellet, D., Constantinesco, A. (1988): Is anti-alpha-fetoprotein immunoscintigraphy a promising approach for the diagnosis of hepatoma? Eur. J. Nucl. Med. 14:612–620.

Dykes, P.W., Hine, K.R., Bradwell, A.R., Blackburn, J.C., Reeder, T.A., Drolc, Z., Booth, S.N. (1980): Localisation of tumour deposits by external scanning after injection of radiolabelled anti-carcinoembryonic antigen. Br. Med. J. 280:220–220.

Epenetos, A.A., Britton, K.E., Mather, S., Shepherd, J., Granowska, M., Taylor-Papadimitriou, J., Nimmon, C.C., Durbin, H., Hawkins, L.R., Malpas, J.S., Bodmer, W.F. (1982): Targeting of iodine-123-labelled tumour-associated monoclonal antibodies to ovarian, breast and gastrointestinal tumours. Lancet 2:999–1006.

Epenetos, A.A., Carr, D., Johnson, P.M., Bodmer, W.F., Lavender, J.P. (1986): Antibody guided radiolocalisation of tumours in patients with testicular or ovarian cancer using two radioiodinated monoclonal antibodies to placental alkaline phosphatase. Br. J. Radiol. 59:117–125.

Esteban, J.M., Colcher, D., Sugarbaker, P., Carrasquillo, J.A., Bryant, G., Thor, A., Reynolds, J.C., Larson, S.M., Schlom, J. (1987): Quantitative and qualitative aspects of radiolocalisation in colon cancer patients of intravenously administered MAB B72.3. Int. J. Cancer 39:50–59.

Farrands, P.A., Perkins, A.C., Pimm, M.V., Hardy, J.G., Baldwin, R.W., Hardcastle, J.D. (1982): Radioimmunodetection of human colorectal cancers using an anti-tumour monoclonal antibody. Lancet 2:397–400.

Gold, P., Freedman, S.E. (1965): Demonstration of tumour specific antigen in human colonic carcinomata by immunological tolerance and absorption techniques. J. Exp. Med. 121:439–462.

Goldenberg, D., DeLand, F.H. (1982): History and status of tumour imaging with radiolabelled antibodies. J. Biol. Response Med. 1:121–136.

Goldenberg, D.M., DeLand, F., Kim, E.E., Bennett, S., Primus, J.J., Van Nagell, J.R., Estes, B., DeSimone, P., Rayburn, P. (1978): Use of radiolabelled antibodies to carcinoembryonic antigen for the detection and localisation of diverse cancers by external photoscanning. N. Engl. J. Med. 298:1384–1388.

Goldenberg, D.M., Kim, E.E., Bennett, S.J., Nelson, M.O., DeLand, F.H. (1983): Carcinoembryonic antigen radioimmunodetection in the evaluation of colorectal cancer and in the detection of occult neoplasms. Gastroenterology 84:524–532.

Granowska, M., Jass, J.R., Britton, K.E., Northover, J.M.A. (1989): A prospective study of the use of 111In-labelled monoclonal antibody against carcino-embryonic antigen in colorectal cancer and of some biological factors affecting its uptake. Int. J. Colorect. Dis. 4:97–108.

Granowska, M., Shepherd, J., Britton, K.E., Ward, B., Mather, S., Taylor-Papadimitriou, J., Epenetos, A.A., Carroll, M.J., Nimmon, C.C., Hawkins, L.A., Slevin, M., Flatman, W., Horne, T., Burchell, V., Durbin, H., Bodmer, W. (1984): Ovarian cancer diagnosis using 123–I monoclonal antibody in comparison with surgical findings. Nucl. Med. Commun. 485–499.

Hertel, A., Baum, R.P., Bosslet, K., Mondorf, U., Hechler, P., Schwartz, A., Bergmann, L., Hor, G. (1990): First use of a Tc-99m labelled monoclonal antibody against the T-cell receptor for the immunoscintigraphic diagnosis of transplant rejection. Eur. J. Nucl. Med. 16:427 (Abstract).

Hui, K.Y., Haber, E., Matsueda, G.R. (1983): Monoclonal antibodies to a synthetic fibrin-like peptide bind to human fibrin but not fibrinogen. Science 222:1129–1132.

Hui, K.Y., Haber, E., Matsueda, G.R. (1985): Immunodetection of human fibrin using monoclonal antibody-64C5 in an extracorporeal chicken model. Thromb. Haemost. 54:524–527.

Johnson, L.L., Sedin, D.W. (1989): The role of antimyosin antibodies in acute myocardial infarction. Semin. Nucl. Med. 19:238–246.

Joseph, K., Hoffken, H., Bosslet, K., Scho-lemmer, H.U. (1988): In vivo labelling of granulocytes with Tc-99m anti-NCA monoclonal antibodies for imaging inflammation. Eur. J. Nucl. Med. 14:367–373.

Keenan, A.M., Harbert, J.C., Larson, S.M. (1985): Monoclonal antibodies in nuclear medicine. J. Nucl. Med. 26:531–537.

Kim, E.E., Deland, F.H., Casper, S., Corgan, R.L., Primus, F.J., Goldenberg, D.M. (1980): Radioimmunodetection of colorectal cancer. Cancer 45: 1243–1247.

Knight, L.C. (1988): Imaging thrombi with radiolabelled anti-fibrin monoclonal antibodies. Nucl. Med. Commun. 9:823–829.

Koblik, P.D., De Nardo, G.L., Berger, H.J. (1989): Current status of immunoscintigraphy in the detection of thrombosis and thromboembolism. Semin. Nucl. Med. (XIX) 3:221–237.

Kudryk, B., Rohoza, A., Ahadi, M., Chin, J., Wiebe, M.E. (1984): Specificity of a monoclonal antibody for the NH_2-terminal region of fibrin. Mol. Immunol. 21:89–94.

Legrand, C., Dubernard, V., Kieffer, N., Nurden, A.T. (1988): Use of a monoclonal antibody to measure the surface expression of thrombospondin following platelet activation. Eur. J. Biochem. 171:393–399.

Locher, J.T., Seybold, K., Andres, R.Y., Schubiger, P., Mach, J.P., Buchegger, F. (1986): Imaging of inflammatory and infectious lesions after injection of radioiodinated monoclonal anti-granulocyte antibodies. Nucl. Med. Commun. 7:659–670.

Mach, J.P., Buchegger, F., Forinini, M., Ritschard, T., Berche, C., Lumbroso, J-D., Mehrege, M., Giracet, C., Accolla, R.S., Carrel, S. (1981): Use of radiolabelled monoclonal anti-CEA antibodies for the detection of human carcinomas by external photoscanning and tomoscintigraphy. Immunol. Today 2:239–249.

Mach, J.P., Chatal, J.F., Lumbroso, J.D., Buchegger, F., Forni, M., Ritschard, J., Berche, C., Douillard, J.Y., Carrel, S., Herlyn, M., Steplewski, Z., Koprowski, H. (1983): Tumour localisation in patients by radiolabelled monoclonal antibodies against colon carcinoma. Cancer Res. 43:5593–5600.

Massuger, R., Classens, R., Verheijen, R., Poels, L., Shijf, C., Hoesel, Q., Corstens, F., Kenemans, P. (1989): Immunoscintigraphy with a new In-111-labelled monoclonal antibody (OV-TL3). Eur. J. Nucl. Med. 15:C1 (Abstract).

Mathieu, A., Lumbroso, J., Bergmann, J.F., Bellet, D., Caillaud, J.M., Baldegrou, P., Struger, M.C., Bohuon, C., Parmintier, C. (1984): Immunoscintigraphy in human squamous lung cancer using monoclonal antibodies. Behring Inst. Mitt. 74:72–79.

McEver, R.P., Martin, M.N. (1984): A monoclonal antibody to a membrane glycoprotein binds only to activated platelets. J. Biol. Chem. 259:9799–9804.

Oster, Z.H., Srivastava, S.C., Som, P., Meiken, G.E., Scudder, L.E., Yamamoto, Y., Atkins, H.L., Brill, A.B., Coller, B.S. (1985): Thrombus radioimmunoscintigraphy: An approach using monoclonal antiplatelet antibody. Proc. Natl. Acad. Sci. USA 82:3465–3468.

Oyen, W.J.G., Claessens, R.A.M.J., van Horn, J.R., van der Meer, J.W.M., Corstens, F.H.M. (1989): Scintigraphic detetion of bone and joint infections with indium-111-labelled nonspecific polyclonal human immunoglobulin G. J. Nucl. Med. 31:403–412.

Palabrica, T.M., Furie, B.C., Konstam, M.A., Aronovitz, M.J., Connolly, R., Brockway, B.A., Rambery, K.L., Furie, B. (1989): Thrombus imaging in a primate model with anti-PADGEM antibodies specific for activated platelets. Proc. Natl. Acad. Sci. USA 86:1036–1040.

Pateisky, N., Philipp, K., Skodler, W.D., Czerwenka, K., Hamilton, G., Burchell, J. (1985): Radioimmunodetection in patients with suspected ovarian cancer. J. Nucl. Med. 26:1369–1376.

Perkins, A.C., Berridge, D.C., Wastie, M.L., Frier, M., Lonsdale, R.J., Makin, G.S., Hopkinson, B.R. (1990): Localisation and assessment of acute peripheral arterial thrombi using platelet specific monoclonal antibody (P256Fab'). Eur. J. Nucl. Med. 16:427 (Abstract).

Perkins, A.C., Pimm, M.V., Gie, C., Marksman, R.A., Symonds, E.M., Baldwin, R.W. (1989): Intraperitoneal ^{131}I- and ^{111}In-791T/36 monoclonal antibody in recurrent ovarian cancer: Imaging and biodistribution. Nucl. Med. Commun. 10:577–584.

Perkins, A.C., Powell, M.C., Wastie, M.L., Scott, I.V., Hitchcock, A., Worthington, B.S., Symonds, E.M. (1990): A prospective evaluation of OC125 and magnetic resonance imaging in patients with ovarian carcinoma. Eur. J. Nucl. Med. 16:311–316.

Perkins, A.C., Whalley, D.R., Ballantyne, K.C., Pimm, M.V. (1988): Gamma camera emission tomography using radiolabelled antibodies. Eur. J. Nucl. Med. 14:45–49.

Perlman, S.B., Folts, J.D., Hammes, R.J., Besozzi, M.C., Mosher, D.F. (1987): The accumulation of a platelet protein, thrombospondin, at the site of arterial thrombus formation: Preliminary report. Eur. J. Nucl. Med. 12:492–495.

Peters, A.M., Lavender, J.P., Needham, S.G., Loutfi, I., Snook, D., Epenetos, A.A., Lumley, P., Keery, R.J., Hogg, N. (1986): Imaging thrombus with radiolabelled monoclonal antibody to platelets. Br. Med. J. 293:1525–1527.

Powell, M.C., Perkins, A.C., Pimm, M.V., Jetaily, M.A.L., Wastie, M.L., Durrant, L., Baldwin, R.W., Symonds, E.M. (1987): Diagnostic imaging of gynecologic tumours with monoclonal antibody 791T/36. Am. J. Obstet. Gynecol. 137:28–34.

Price, M.R., Pimm, M.V., Page, C.M., Armitage, N.C., Hardcastle, J.D., Baldwin, R.W. (1984): Immunolocalisation of the murine monoclonal antibody 791T/36 within primary human colorectal carcinomas and identification of the target antigen. Br. J. Cancer 49:809–812.

Rainsbury, R.M., Ott, R.J., Westwood, J.H., Kalirai, T.S., Coombes, R.C., McCready, V.R., Neville, A.M., Gazet, J.C. (1983): Location of metastatic breast carcinoma by a monoclonal antibody chelate labelled with In-111. Lancet 2:934–938.

Richardson, R.B., Davies, A.G., Bourne, S.P., Staddon, G.E., Jones, D.H., Kemshed, J.T., Coakham, H.B. (1986): Radioimmunolocalisation of human brain tumours: Biodistribution of radiolabelled monoclonal antibody UJ13A. Eur. J. Nucl. Med. 12:313–320.

Rosebrough, S.F., Kudryk, B., Grossman, Z.D., McAfee, J.G., Subrumanian, G., Ritter-Hrncirik, C.A., Witanowski, L.S., Tillapaugh-Fay, G. (1985): Radioimmunoimaging of venous thrombi using iodine-131 monoclonal antibody. Radiology 156:515–517.

Rosebrough, S.F., Grossman, Z.D., McAfee, J.G., Kudryk, B.J., Subrumanian, G., Ritter-Hrncirik, C.A., Witanowski, L.S., Tillapaugh-Fay, G., Urritia, E. (1987): Aged venous thrombi: Radioimmunoimaging with fibrin-specific monoclonal antibody. Radiology 162:575–577.

Rosebrough, S.F., Grossman, Z.D., McAfee, J.G., Kudryk, B.J., Subrumanian, G., Ritter-Hrncirck, C.A., Witanowski, L.S., Tillapaugh-Fay, G., Urritia, E., Zapf-Longo, C. (1988): Thrombus imaging with indium-111 and iodine-131-labelled fibrin-specific monoclonal antibody and its F(ab')$_2$ and Fab fragments. J. Nucl. Med. 29:1212–1222.

Ryan, K.P., Dillman, R.O., DeNardo, S.J., DeNardo, G.L., Beauregard, J., Hagan, P.L., Amox, D.G., Clutter, M.L., Burnett, K.G., Rulot, C.M., Sobol, R.E., Abramson, A., Bartholomew, R.K., Frincke, J.M., Birdwell, C.R., Carlo, D.J., O'Grady, L.F., Halpern, S.E. (1988): Breast cancer imaging with In-111 human IgM monoclonal antibodies: Preliminary studies. Radiology 167:71–75.

Rylatt, D.B., Blake, A.S., Cottis, L.E., Massingham, D.A., Fletcher, W.A., Masci, P.P., Whitaker, A.N., Elms, M., Bunce, I., Webber, A.J., Wyatt, D., Bundesen, P.G. (1983): An immunoassay for human D dimer using monoclonal antibodies. Thromb. Res. 31:767–768.

Scheefers-Borchel, U., Muller-Berghaus, G., Fuhge, P., Eberle, R., Heimberger, N. (1985): Discrimination between fibrin and fibrinogen by a monoclonal antibody against a synthetic peptide. Proc. Natl. Acad. Sci. USA 82:7091–7095.

Scheidhauer, K., Markl, A., Leinsinger, G., Moser, E., Scheiffarth, O.F., Riedel, K.G., Schaal, T.S., Stefani, F.H., Schumacher, U. (1988): Immunoscintigraphy in intraocular malignant melanoma. Nucl. Med. Commun. 9:669–679.

Schwarz, A., Steinstraesser, A. (1987): A novel approach to Tc-99m-labelled monoclonal antibodies. J. Nucl. Med. 28:721 (Abstract).

Sfakianakis, G.N., DeLand, F.H. (1982): Radioimmunodiagnosis and radioimmunotherapy. J. Nucl. Med. 23:840–850.

Som, P., Oster, Z.H., Zamora, P.O., Yamamoto, K., Sacker, D.F., Brill, A.B., Newell, K.D., Rhodes, B.A. (1986): Radioimmunoimaging of experimental thrombi in dogs using technetium-99m-labelled monoclonal antibody fragments reactive with human platelets. J. Nucl. Med. 27:1315–1320.

Stenberg, P.E., McEver, R.P., Shuman, M.A., Jacques, Y.V., Bainton, D.F. (1985): A platelet alpha-granule membrane protein (GMP-140) is expressed on the plasma membrane after activation. J. Cell Biol. 101:880–886.

Stuttle, A.W.J., Klosok, J., Peters, A.M., Lavender, J.P. (1989): Sequential imaging of post-operative thrombus using the In-111-labelled platelet-specific monoclonal antibody P256. Br. J. Radiol. 62:963–969.

Stuttle, A.W.J., Ritter, J.M., Peters, A.M., Lavender, J.P. (1988): In vitro studies with an antiplatelet monoclonal antibody; P256. Nucl. Med. Commun. 9:813–815.

Symonds E.M., Perkins, A.C., Pimm, M.V., Baldwin, R.W., Hardy, J.G., Williams, D.A. (1985): Clinical implications for immunoscintigraphy in patients with ovarian malignancy: A preliminary study using monoclonal antibody 791T/36. Br. J. Obs. Gynaecol. 92: 270–276.

Thakur, M.L. (1988): Potential of radiolabeled antiplatelet antibodies in the detection of vascular thrombi. In: Srivastava SC (ed.): Radiolabeled Monoclonal Antibodies for Imaging and Therapy, NATO ASI Series A: Life Sciences, vol 152. Plenum: New York, pp 831–842.

Thakur, M.L., Richard, M.D., White III, F.W. (1988): Monoclonal antibodies as agents for selective radiolabeling of human neutrophils. J. Nucl. Med. 29: 1817–1825.

Thakur, M.L., Thiagarajan, P., White III, F., Park, C.H., Maurer, P.H. (1987): Monoclonal antibodies for specific cell labelling: consideration, preparation and preliminary evaluation. Nucl. Med. Biol. 14:51–58.

Tjandra, J.J., Russell, I.S., Collins, J.P., Andrews, J.T., Lichtenstein, M., Binns, D., McKenzie, I.F.C. (1989): Immunolymphoscintigraphy for the detection of lymph node metastases from breast cancer. Cancer Res. 49:1600–1608.

Future Developments and Clinical Prospects in Immunoscintigraphy

FUTURE DEVELOPMENTS IN IMMUNOSCINTIGRAPHY

In addition to the continuing development of new monoclonal antibodies and methods for their radiolabelling, other approaches to the use of antibodies in immunoscintigraphy are being investigated. These are aimed particularly at increasing the relatively low target to non-target ratios achievable at the present time with monoclonal antibodies and at reducing their immunogenicity, so that repeated investigations can be feasible on a routine basis.

Increasing Target to Non-Target Ratios

Pre-targeted immunoscintigraphy. The low target to non-target ratios usually achieved with antibodies is due not only to the low absolute amount of antibody accumulating in the target tissue, but also to the relatively long blood pool survival of remaining radiolabelled material. One proposed method to overcome this problem is to administer the antibody, without a radiolabel, and then when it has accumulated in target tissue, but blood-pool background levels have dropped, a radiolabelled tracer capable of binding to the antibody is injected. This method, where antibody alone is targeted first, is termed pre-targetting. Ideally the labelled tracer should show rapid and efficient binding to the pre-targeted antibody, but otherwise be cleared from the blood and catabolized more rapidly than antibody.

Bispecific anti-tumour anti-chelate antibodies. One possibility for pre-targeted immunoscintigraphy is to use a bispecific antibody which can react both with the target tissue antigen and then with a small radiolabelled tracer. Studies in patients with colorectal carcinoma, with a bispecific antibody capable of binding to both CEA and radioindium labelled chelate (benzyl-EDTA), have shown that this approach can work (Stickney et al., 1989). The effect could perhaps be increased if antibody surviving in the blood is cleared by injection of the chelate conjugated to a carrier human protein such as transferrin some hours before labelled chelate alone is given. One problem with this approach is the small amount of chelate, and therefore of radiolabel, which can be captured by the pre-targeted antibody, and there is as yet no published large-scale clinical assessment of its efficiency.

Avidin and biotin conjugated antibodies. An alternative system which is undergoing experimental evaluation is that of using avidin and biotin. Avidin is a protein, of about 70,000 dalton molecular weight, found in egg white, and there is a similar material called streptavidin of microbial origin. These proteins react with extraordinarily high affinity with the small molecular size (244 Da) vitamin biotin, the association constant of this interaction being about 10^{15}, which is four or five orders of magnitude higher than that of antibody–antigen interactions. With this system one approach would be to inject the monoclonal antibody conjugated to biotin, allow maximum accumulation in target tissue to take place, and then inject suitably labelled avidin or streptavidin and image some time later. To prevent the labelled avidin complexing with antibody-biotin still remaining in the circulation, unlabelled avidin could be given some time before the labelled avidin. The complexes formed between the excess biotin-antibody and the unlabelled avidin would probably have been cleared from the circulation by time the labelled avidin was given.

An alternative method would be to give biotinylated antibody, followed by unlabelled avidin or streptavidin, which would partly localise in the biotin bound to the target lesion and partly facilitate clearance of circulating biotinylated antibody. Radiolabelled biotin could then be given to be taken up by the avidin being held in the tumour by the biotin of the initial pre-targeted antibody.

The converse way of using this system would be to conjugate the avidin or streptavidin to the antibody, pre-target this to the target lesion, and then inject radiolabelled biotin. Perhaps here excess antibody-avidin conjugate could be cleared from the circulation by giving biotin conjugated to another protein, such as transferrin.

Although there are a number of reports of experimental investigation of these possibilities (Hnatowich et al., 1987; Pimm et al., 1988; Pagenelli et al., 1988; Oehr et al., 1988) and small clinical trials have been carried out, their clinical application would have several problems. Firstly, avidin and streptavidin alone are cleared rapidly from the circulation, particularly to the kidneys, and these organs certainly tend to dominate images of animals after the injection of I-131- or In-111-labelled preparations. Secondly, avidin and streptavidin are immunogenic, and this could preclude their use in some patients who may be sensitive to egg proteins and/or in repeat investigations. Thirdly, because biotin, being a vitamin, is naturally present in human blood and tissues, either the natural role of this material may be perturbed by injection of avidin or the intended distribution of the labelled avidin or the avidin-antibody conjugate may be affected by the endogenous biotin.

Bispecific antibodies against dual tumour-associated antigens. The use of mixtures of two antibodies, each against a different antigen, either or both of which may possibly be present in a target lesion, will not actually increase target to non-target ratios in the final images, because blood levels and normal organ levels of the radiolabel will also be increased. But if a single antibody can react with two different antigens, then potentially target to non-target ratios can be increased.

Hybridoma technology has developed to the production of quadromas which can be used to generate such hybrid antibodies, one combining site of which recognises one antigen, and the other combining site of which recognises another antigen. This method can be used to produce monoclonal antibodies reacting with two different tumour-associated antigens co-expressed on the same tumour cells. Bosslet et al. (1989), have reported the production of such a hybrid monoclonal antibody reacting with both CEA and another different antigen associated with gastrointestinal cancer.

Although there are not yet reports of imaging with these types of antibodies, it is expected that they could increase the sensitivity of immunoscintigraphy and increase the absolute amount of antibody localising per unit weight of tumour tissue.

Alternative antibody fragments.
Antibody fragments which have been evaluated both experimentally and clinically for immunoscintigraphy have been $F(ab')_2$ and Fab. The rationale for the use of these fragments is that they pass out from the blood into extravascular fluid more quickly and to a greater extent, speeding up target localisation, and they are catabolised far more rapidly than intact antibody so that blood backgrounds are lower. Their major disadvantages are that rapid catabolism reduces the absolute amount localising in target tissue, and catabolism in and excretion through the kidneys can mean that these dominate abdominal images, particularly with radiometal-labelled antibodies.

Several other types of antibody fragments can be produced by appropriate enzyme digestion of monoclonal antibodies, and these might be worth evaluation for immunoscintigraphy. For example, Fab/c fragments of the 791T/36 monoclonal antibody have been reported to give somewhat greater and faster extravasation than the intact antibody and to localise in tumour xenografts (Demignot et al., 1990). These fragments have only one Fab site but an intact Fc part. How efficiently these sort of fragments may be at tumour imaging has yet to be assessed.

Genetically engineered antibody fragments.
As an alternative to the production of antibody fragments from existing monoclonal antibodies by chemical methods, the techniques of genetic engineering are also now able to produce antibody fragments (Morrison and Oi, 1990; Rodwell, 1989). Using genetic engineering techniques, the production of small fragment-like components of antibodies, actually grown in bacteria rather than in hybridoma cells, has recently been reported.

The binding of an antibody to its antigen requires interaction of combining sites on both the heavy and light chains. Constructs consisting of these two variable region combining sites, and therefore termed *Fv fragments,* can be engineered with the same antigen binding characteristics as the antibody from which it was derived.

Although with many antibodies, binding to antigen depends upon the complementing effect of the heavy and light chain, at least in some situations the heavy-chain variable region alone seems to have an affinity for antigen approaching that of intact antibody. Using genetic engineering methods, it is possible to produce small molecules consisting essentially of just the variable part of the heavy chain of the antibody. Because they are just a single part, or domain, of the antibody binding site, they are being termed single domain antibodies or dAb's (Ward et al., 1989).

Although not yet reported to tumour-associated or other antigens of interest in immunoscintigraphy, it will probably be feasible to produce such Fv fragments and also dAb's. Their potential advantages lie in their small size, giving potentially good and rapid tissue penetration, with rapid clearance from the blood, and probably rapid catabolism, although their biodistribution has not yet been assessed. In addition, they would probably be much less immunogenic than intact antibodies or conventional fragments.

Decreasing Immune Responses to Monoclonal Antibodies

The fact that virtually all monoclonal antibody hitherto used for immunoscintigraphy are of murine origin means that their is the possibility, or rather probability, of them inducing immune responses in the patients.

If human monoclonal antibodies could be used instead, this would overcome many of the problems of immunogenicity. However, the production of wholly human monoclonal antibodies has always proved difficult. This is because the generation of such antibodies requires the target antigen to be immunogenic in the person from whom lymphocytes for fusion to generate the hybridoma are derived. This is very unlikely with target antigens which occur naturally such as fibrin or platelet antigens, and not very likely with antigens associated with tumours.

Although a few human monoclonal antibodies have been reported to tumours, the greatest interest at present is in the generation, by genetic engineering techniques, of "chimeric" antibodies in which much of the original mouse immunoglobulin molecule has been replaced with human immunoglobulin, leaving only parts of the heavy and light chains which contain the binding site of the original murine antibody. In some cases it is possible to introduce into a human immunoglobulin only the combin-

ing sites of the mouse antibody, giving an even more human-like antibody, termed a *humanised antibody*.

Such antibodies are now being produced to a number of antigens of interest in tumour immunoscintigraphy such as CEA (Hardman et al., 1989) and the antigen defined by the B72.3 monoclonal antibody (Colcher et al., 1989). Their use in patients, vis-à-vis efficiency in imaging tumours and lack of immunogenicity, has yet to be reported, but if these are favourable, it can be envisaged that other monoclonal antibodies will be similarly "chimerised" or "humanised."

CLINICAL PROSPECTS

The continued growth of the speciality of nuclear medicine depends upon advances in both equipment and technology. The clinical use of antibody-based radiopharmaceuticals has already regenerated a great deal of enthusiasm for nuclear medicine techniques, and these products are becoming generally accepted, although there is still some resistance to their widespread application. Patient studies have generally been performed in specialised centres with local expertise in this field of work. However, we are now at a stage when Tc-99m antibodies can be prepared in the radiopharmacy as easily as any other radiopharmaceutical (immunoscintigraphy has finally matured). The main problems remaining over the use of antibodies at the present time are those of availability, specificity, adverse reactions, and cost. Despite the relatively long list of antibodies given in the Appendix: Antibody Look Up Table, this volume, relatively few have been taken up by commercial concerns.

The role of immunoscintigraphy in clinical oncology appears to be restricted to monitoring patients with recurrent disease, but it is the non-oncological application which would appear to be clinically most promising. We are currently witnessing the introduction of antibodies specific for circulating cells, parasites, and microorganisms. The production of antibodies specific for cells in the circulation offers a convenient means of radiolabelling without affecting cell function. Antibodies directed against parasites would be of great value in the diagnosis of a range of life-threatening conditions. The production of new antibodies and fragments coupled with more exact dosing regimens (Thomas et al., 1990) to suit the patients condition will undoubtedly improve the performance of the technique, leading to more widespread clinical acceptance.

Currently, the marketing of monoclonal antibodies is being inhibited by regulatory restrictions, and licensing of products is becoming prohibitively expensive. Production techniques are becoming more closely monitored, and documentation is required for each and every step taken leading to the final product. It is interesting to note that the guidelines on the production of antibodies from cell supernatants rather than from ascites fluid originated as much from animal rights campaigners as from the desire to limit viral contamination of the product. There is no question regarding the need for safeguarding the efficiency of antibodies administered to patients, but there is an overwhelming need for the widespread availability of inexpensive radiopharmaceutical products which will ultimately benefit patients. Even at the present time, the number of adverse reactions for murine monoclonal antibodies is no greater than those reported from the use of radiological contrast media.

Further refinements to the technique of immunoscintigraphy will undoubtedly evolve. We are already seeing the *in vivo* use of human-mouse chimeric antibodies labelled with I-124 and imaged with positron emission tomography (PET) (Westera et al., 1990). As technology progresses, this type of study will become commonplace. Hopefully, the patient will be the final beneficiary.

REFERENCES AND FURTHER READING

Bosslet, K., Schwarz, A., Steinstrasser, A., Seidel, L., Sedlacek, H.H. (1989): Bispecific anti-CEA-anti-mucin monoclonal antibody for immunoscintigraphy of gastrointestinal tract carcinomas. Eur. J. Nucl. Med. 15:C4.

Colcher, D., Milenic, D., Roselli, M., Raubitschek, A., Yarranton, G., King, D., Adair, J., Whittle, N., Bodmer, M., Schlom, J. (1989): Characterization and biodistribution of recombinant and recombinant/chimeric constructs of monoclonal antibody B72.3. Cancer Res. 49:1738–1745.

Demignot, S., Pimm, M.V., Baldwin, R.W. (1990): Comparison of biodistribution of 791T/36 monoclonal antibody and its Fab/c fragment in BALB/c mice and nude mice bearing human tumour xenografts. Cancer Res. 50:2936–2942.

Dick, H.M. (1990): Single domain antibodies. Br. Med. Journal 300: 959–960.

Hardman, N., Gill, L.L., De Winter, R.F.J., Wagner, K., Hollis, M., Businger, F., Ammaturo, D., Buchegger, F., Mach, J-P., Heusser, C. (1989): Generation of a recombinant mouse-human chimaeric monoclonal antibody directed against human carcinoembryonic antigen. Int. J. Cancer 44:424–433.

Hnatowich, D.J., Virzi, F., Rusckowsi, M. (1987): Investigations of avidin and biotin for imaging applications. J. Nucl. Med. 28:1294–1302.

Morrison, S.L., Oi, V.T. (1990): Genetically engineered antibody molecules. Adv. Immunol. 44:65–92.

Oehr, P., Wesretman, J., Biersack, H.J. (1988): Streptavidin and biotin as potential tumour imaging agents. J. Nucl. Med. 29:728–729.

Paganelli, G., Riva, P., Deleide, G., Clivio, A., Chiolerio, F., Scassellati, G.A., Malcovati, M., Siccardi, A.G. (1988): *In vivo* labelling of biotinylated monoclonal antibodies by radioactive avidin: a strategy to increase tumor radiolocalization. Int. J. Cancer Suppl. 2:121–125.

Pimm, M.V., Fells, H.F., Perkins, A.C., Baldwin, R.W. (1988): Iodine-131 and indium-111 labelled avidin and streptavidin for pre-targeted immunoscintigraphy with biotinylated anti-tumour monoclonal antibody. Nucl. Med. Commun. 9:931–941.

Rodwell, J.D. (1989): Engineering monoclonal antibodies. Nature 342:99–100.

Rogan, M.T., Morris, D.L., Pritchard, D.I., Perkins, A.C. (1990): Echinococcus granulosus: the potential use of specific radiolabelled antibodies in diagnosis by immunoscintigraphy. Clin. Exp. Immunol. 80:225–231.

Stickney, D.R., Slater, J.B., Kirk, G.A., Ahlem, C., Chang, C-H., Frincke, J.M. (1989): Bifunctional antibody: ZCH/CHA indium-111 BLEDTA-IV clinical imaging in colorectal carcinoma. Antibody, Immunoconjugates, and Radiopharmaceuticals 2:1–14.

Thomas, G.D., Chappell, M.J., Dykes, P.W., Ramsden, D.B., Godfrey, K.R., Ellis, J.R.M., Bradwell, A.R. (1990): Effect of dose, molecular size, affinity, and protein binding on tumour uptake of antibody ligand: A biomathematical model. Cancer Res. 49:3290–3296.

Ward, E., Gussow, D., Griffiths, A.D., Jones, P.T., Winter, G. (1989): Binding activities of a repertoire of single immunoglobulin variable domains secreted from Escherichia coli. Nature 341:544–546.

Westera, G., Reist, H.W., Buchegger, F., Pfeiffer, A., Van Schulthes, G.K., Weinreich, R., Mach, J.P. (1990): Positron emission tomography in colon tumour radioimmuno imaging using a I-124-labelled anti-CEA monoclonal antibody (MAB). Eur. J. Nucl. Med. 16:393 (Abstract).

Glossary of Immunological Terms

Affinity chromatography. A technique for isolating antibodies. Antigen is attached chemically to an inert support medium and usually packed into a long narrow column. Antibody solution is run through, the antibody is absorbed by the antigen, and is subsequently eluted off, usually by reduction of the pH. The same technique is used with other materials capable of absorbing antibody, such as Protein A.

Affinity. A measure of the strength of binding of an antibody to antigen. This can be quantified as an affinity constant, more correctly called the equilibrium constant. (See antigen-antibody binding.)

Agglutination reactions. These can be used to detect either antigen or antibody naturally occurring on, or artificially attached to, the surface of particles such as red blood cells or latex particles. The particles are agglutinated because of their being cross-linked by antibody or antigen.

Allotype. Variations due to genetic differences within a species.

Allograft. A graft of tissue between individuals of the same species.

Antibody. A protein, the production of which is stimulated by contact with a for-eign material, the antigen. Antibodies can bind specifically to the antigen which induced their formation.

Antibody affinity. A measure of the strength of the bond formed between an antibody and an antigen. Strictly, this term refers to the bonding between a single antibody-combining site and a single antigenic determinant, and avidity is a measure of the multivalent interaction of antibody and antigen. It is dependent on a balance between various non-covalent interactions, attracting the paratope of the antibody to the epitope of the antigen and any repulsive forces created between their electron clouds. The affinity of an antibody for antigen is measured *in vitro* by determining the amounts of bound and free antigen and antibody when mixed together, and using analyses such as Scatchard plots.

Antigen-antigen binding. These are non-covalent binding reactions dependent upon the structural relationship between the molecules. Three main forces are involved: coulombic attraction, hydrogen bonding, and Van der Waals forces. Equilibrium is reached when the rate of association of the antibody and antigen is equalled by the rate of dissociation of the complex. The equilibrium constant $K_e = K_a/K_d$

= [AbAg]/[Ab][Ag], where K_a and K_d are the association and dissociation constants. Concentrations have to be measured in molar terms, and the units for K_e are litres/mole.

Antibody classes. There are a number of different classes of antibody, differing in the nature of their heavy chains and each with different natural biological functions. In immunoscintigraphy those of the IgG and IgM classes are of most interest and importance.

Antibody-combining site. That structure present on an antibody molecule which combines with the antigen.

Antibody fragments. Antibodies can be broken down by enzymes (particularly pepsin and papain), and/or reduction of the disulphide bonds holding the antibody chains together, into fragments. Those of most importance in immunoscintigraphy are the Fab and F(ab')$_2$ fragments of IgG antibodies. Fab fragments have a molecular weight of 50,000 daltons and only one combining site; F(ab')$_2$ fragments are 100,000 daltons and have two combining sites. Fab fragments are usually produced by papain digestion of the antibody, and F(ab')$_2$ by pepsin digestion, although papain digestion can be used with some IgG isotypes to give what should strictly be described as F(ab)$_2$ fragments. Both lack the Fc portion of the original antibody molecule and therefore have a much altered biodistribution. IgM antibodies can also be fragmented, to a so-called monomeric form, which is produced by breaking the bonds holding together the five subunits of the intact pentameric molecule, and the monomers can be further fragmented into F(ab')$_2$ and Fab type subunits.

Antibody response. The induction and development of antibodies in response to antigen. In the present context two types of responses are important. One is the response produced by deliberate immu-nization, usually of mice, with an antigen as part of the process of monoclonal antibody production. The other is the deleterious response against the monoclonal antibody itself in patients given monoclonal antibody. For the latter sort, various terms are given to the different types of responses, such as HAMA (human anti-mouse antibody) and HAHA (human anti-human antibody).

Antibody valency. This refers to the number of binding sites on an antibody molecule. IgG antibodies and their F(ab')$_2$ fragments have two combining sites, and are bivalent. Fab fragments of IgG antibodies have one combining site and are mono- or uni-valent. IgM antibodies have ten combining sites.

Antigen. A substance against which an immune response can be evoked. Such substances are often termed immunogenic.

Anti-idiotypic antibody (ANTI-id). An antibody which reacts with that part of another antibody molecule which is meant to react with its own antigen. Such antibodies can prevent binding of the second antibody to its target.

Bispecific antibody. An antibody whose two combining sites react with different antigens. Also called hybrid antibodies.

CEA (carcinoembryonic antigen). A glycoprotein expressed on foetal endodermal tissue and re-expressed in some adult malignant cells, particularly colorectal carcinoma. It was one of the first target antigens for immunoscintigraphy, and a range of monoclonal antibodies have now been produced to a number of different epitopes on the molecule.

Chimeric antibody. Antibodies containing components derived from two different species of animals. Those of interest for immunoscintigraphy contain mainly human immunoglobulin structures, but with the combining site derived from mouse or rat antibody against the antigen of interest. The advantage of such antibodies is that they have the target recognition capability of the murine antibody, but being composed mainly of human immunoglobulin, they will probably evoke little adverse reactions in patients.

Chromatography. Originally demonstrated as a technique for separation and purification of materials which were readily identified by their different colours, the term is now used for a wide variety of biochemical separation techniques. Affinity chromatography and gel filtration chromatography are the most widely used in the purification and study of antibodies.

Clone. A population of cells which have been produced by growth and division of a single parent cell.

Cloning. The technique of isolation of a single cell (usually *in vitro*) which can then be grown up into a clonal population.

DTPA Diethylenetriaminepentacetic acid. This is a chelating agent widely used to attach radiometals to antibodies. The anhydride of the material is reacted first with the antibody.

ELISA (enzyme-linked immunosorbent assay). This is a widely used method for detecting and quantifying antibodies, particularly monoclonal antibodies. Usually target antigen is adsorbed to a solid phase, and then antibody, such as mouse monoclonal antibody, is applied. Its binding to the antigen is then detected by a subsequent reaction with anti-mouse Ig antibody which has been conjugated to an enzyme, usually peroxidase or a phosphatase. The presence of the enzyme-conjugated antibody is detected by addition of an appropriate chromogenic substrate, which is acted upon by the enzyme to give a coloured product which can be measured by its absorbance of light in a spectrophotometer.

Epitope. The actual site within an antigen that is recognized by the combining site of an antibody. There may be more than one, and sometimes multiple epitopes on one antigen molecule.

Gel filtration chromatography. An analytical and preparative technique widely used in the study of antibodies in which antibody molecules, fragments, etc., are separated by passage through porous solid media with pores of the size of the molecules under study, thus achieving a form of filtration at the molecular level.

Heavy and light chains. Antibody molecules are made up of two types of subunits. There are five different types of heavy chain, corresponding to the five classes of immunoglobulin, those of IgG and IgM being designated as γ and μ, respectively, and having molecular weight of 50,000 and 70,000 daltons, respectively. There are two types of light chain, termed *kappa* and *lambda*. Each IgG molecule is made of two identical heavy (H) chains and two identical light (L) chains. IgM molecules have five IgG-like units linked together by a J chain.

Humanisation. Most monoclonal antibodies currently available are of murine origin. The antigen-combining sites of these antibodies can be genetically engineered into human immunoglobulins to give chimeric antibodies. This process is sometimes called *humanisation,* although the resulting monoclonal antibody is not really fully human.

HPLC (high-performance liquid chromatography). A chromatographic technique which can be used for analysis of proteins such as antibodies. It is faster and more sensitive than many other chromatographic techniques but requires more specialised equipment and expertise.

Hybridoma. A hybrid cell produced by a physical fusion of two different cells. Hybridomas produced by fusing myeloma cells with spleen cells from animals immunized with appropriate antigen are used to produce monoclonal antibodies.

Hybrid antibody. An antibody whose two combining sites react with different antigens. They can be constructed either by fragmentation of two existing antibodies and chemical re-association of the Fab containing part of one antibody with the Fab part of the other, or by fusion of two existing hybridomas, each producing different monoclonal antibodies.

Hypersensitivity. A general term for any exaggerated immune response. There are a number of types with different mechanisms and consequences. Those which may occasionally occur in patients given antibodies for immunoscintigraphy are of the immediate type. One form is caused by the patient's production of IgE antibodies to the antibody being used for immunoscintigraphy. These antibodies are predominantly tissue-bound antibodies and on contact with the antigen (i.e., the imaging antibody) cause local release of intermediates, which causes anaphylactic shock with marked vasodilation, leakage of intravascular fluid, and bronchoconstriction. The other is due to high levels of circulating antibodies (particularly IgG antibodies) which form immune complexes with the intravenously given imaging antibody. These complexes can cause nephritis and arteritis.

Idiotypes. The idiotope of an antibody is that part of the combining site which combines with antigen. Strictly, it is the paratope which is the actual specific combining site.

IgG, IgM. Abbreviations for gamma immunoglobulin and macro-immunoglobulin, the major classes of immunoglobulins and those to which the majority of monoclonal antibodies of interest for immunoscintigraphy belong.

Immune complex. The complex formed when an antigen reacts with antibody. Such complexes can form in the plasma between circulating antigen, released, for example, from tumours, and a monoclonal antibody injected for immunoscintigraphy. These particular form of immune complexes seem to remain in the circulation and do not seem to be detrimental. Other sorts of complexes can form between monoclonal antibody and antibody produced by the patient against the monoclonal antibody. These sorts of complexes do seem to be cleared from the circulation, and this can have detrimental effects on imaging.

Immunoadsorbent. A solid-phase material to which has been chemically linked an antibody or antigen. Used for purification of antibodies or antigens in affinity chromatography.

Immunoconjugate. A combination of an antibody or antibody fragment with a chemical compound intended for linkage to a radionuclide or drug molecule. The term is often used to refer to an antibody-drug conjugate itself, frequently to mean a conjugate to be used therapeutically.

Immunodiffusion. A technique to detect reaction between antibodies and antigen in a soluble form. The antigen and antibody are allowed to diffuse towards one another through gel (usually of agar), and where they meet and combine a visible line of precipitation will occur in the gel. The method can be made quantitative by using ranges of dilutions of antibody or antigen, so that concentrations of unknown antigens can be determined by reference to standards or the titre of antibody determined.

Immunofluorescence. A technique for microscopic localisation of antigen by its reaction with an antibody carrying a fluorescent dye which is visualised by excitation with ultraviolet light.

Immunogenic. Capable of generating an immune response. Immunogenicity is the measure of the degree of ability of a substance to be an immunogen.

Immunoglobulin. Strictly speaking, the globulin fraction of serum which contains antibody activity. But this term is now often used as a synonym for antibody. It is abbreviated to Ig, but this abbreviation is usually extended to IgG, IgM etc., to show the class of immunoglobulin. There are five classes, IgG, IgM, IgA, IgE, and IgD, but the first two are the types most frequently encountered as monoclonal antibodies.

Immunohistology. A technique in which tissue sections or cell smears are "stained" with antibodies to identify antigens recognised by the antibody. This is widely used in screening hybridomas for production of monoclonal antibodies reactive with target tissue but not normal tissues. Generally, tissue is reacted with the antibody of, say, mouse origin, and binding is detected by the subsequent addition of a second antibody to mouse immunoglobulin conjugated to an enzyme. Subsequent addition of the substrate for the enzyme results in generation of coloured product specifically at the site within the tissue where the original monoclonal antibody reacted with its antigen.

Immunoradiopharmaceutical. A radioactive preparation of pharmaceutical quality based on an antibody or antibody fragment which is intended for *in vivo* administration for the purpose of diagnosis or therapy. Such preparations are in the main intended for immunoscintigraphy or immunotherapy.

Immunoscintigraphy. Use of a radiolabelled antibody preparation for imaging with a gamma camera. Sometimes referred to as radioimmunoscintigraphy (RIS) or radioimmunodetection (RAID).

Immunosuppression. The state of having reduced immune responses. Such immunosuppression can be deliberately induced—for example, in transplant pa-

tients. Immunosuppression has been used in patients receiving murine antibody preparations to prevent the formation of anti-mouse antibodies. Most measures are not antigen-specific and involve the use of drugs such as cyclosporin A.

Immunotherapy. The use of an antibody preparation for therapy either by attaching a radionuclide (radioimmunotherapy) or a cytotoxic drug or toxin.

Immunotoxin. An antibody or antibody fragment linked to a cytotoxic agent. The term is usually used for conjugates with toxins other than conventional therapeutic drugs, such as highly toxic plant or bacterial toxins.

Isotype. Variants of immunoglobulins, such as the different antibody classes. Within classes there are also different isotypes. Of particular importance in immunoscintigraphy are the different isotypes of the mouse IgG immunoglobulins, which are the IgG1, IgG2a, IgG2b, and IgG3. These different isotypes differ in the ease in which fragments can be prepared.

Monoclonal antibody. Antibody produced from a clone of antibody-producing cells. The clonal nature of the cells results in all antibody molecules in the preparation being identical in class, isotype, and, antigen-combining properties.

Murine. Derived from animals belonging to the Muridae Family. Although often used to refer to material from mice, the term covers both mice and rats. Thus "monoclonal antibodies of murine origin" could be from either species.

NCA (normal cross-reacting antigen). A CEA-like glycoprotein. It is expressed in normal cells, particularly those of the monocyte and myeloid series. Although some monoclonal antibodies to CEA react only with CEA, others may cross react with NCA. This may cause loss of specificity if these antibodies are used to image CEA-producing tumours.

Nude mice. Nude mice have a genetic defect which results in their having no thymus, and therefore being unable to mount an immune response. They are widely used to grow xenografts of human tumours. A linked genetic defect results in their being hairless; thus their appearance which gave rise to their official name. The nude (nu) gene has been introduced into many inbred strains of mice, and thus homogeneous populations of animals are available for xenograft growth. Nude rats are also available, but have been little used in developing immunoscintigraphy.

Paratope. That part of an antibody which combines with the epitope of an antigen. The paratope is within the epitope, a broader term to describe the region of the antibody containing the combining site.

Passage. The surgical movement of a transplantable tumour from one animal (the donor) to another (the recipient). For example, having established a human tumour as a xenograft in a nude mouse, the tumour can be maintained, virtually indefinitely, by passaging tissue from it periodically into more nude mice. Such passaged human tumour xenografts have been frequently used to examine the localisation of antibodies in tumours.

Polyclonal antibody. Antibody produced from multiple clones of cells. They are rarely produced *in vitro*, and the term usually refers to antibody isolated from serum of animals immunized with antigen. Even after purification, the preparations contain a mixture of antibodies against different antigenic epitopes. Such antibodies are of little use for immunoscintigraphy because of the difficulties in obtaining the required antigen specificity and purity. Exceptions include antibodies to antigens such as CEA, which are available in pure form for immunization and antibody purification.

Protein A. A protein, isolated from *Staphylococcus aureus,* which has the ability to bind to IgG immunoglobulins. Protein A, immobilized onto a suitable solid support, can be used in the purification of immunoglobulins, including monoclonal antibodies. Immunoglobulins bound to the Protein A can be eluted off by low pH buffers or high salt concentrations. Different isotypes of immunoglobulins elute off different pHs, and this method can be used to purify one isotype from another.

Quadroma. The fusion of two hybridomas produces a hybrid of four cell types, sometimes referred to as a quadroma. Such quadromas can be used, for example, to produce bispecific antibodies which react with both of the antigens originally recognised by the two parent hybridomas.

Radioimmunoassay. Quantitative determination of the concentration of an antigen or an antibody involving the detection of one or another of the reactants by virtue of its carrying a radiolabel. In an indirect radioimmunoassay, neither antigen or antibody is labelled, but there is a final detection step with radiolabelled material —for example, labelled anti-mouse IgG antibody to detect a mouse monoclonal antibody.

Scatchard analysis. A method of mathematical analysis of the interaction of two reactants, frequently used to determine the affinity of an antibody for antigen. Antibody at a range of concentrations is reacted with antigen, and the ratio of the concentration of bound antibody to free antibody is plotted against that of bound antibody. The slope of the line is the equilibrium constant K.

Second generation antibodies. Antigens which have been isolated using monoclonal antibody directed against them can then be used to immunise mice to produce a "second generation" of antibodies. Often the antigens recognised by monoclonal antibodies were only originally identified when an antibody was produced against them. The availability of antigen makes the production of further antibodies much less of a hit-or-miss response. The availability of this approach makes much easier the selection of antibodies with more advantageous properties, such as high affinity, ease of fragmentation, etc.

Seed lots. These are samples of hybridoma cells taken soon after cloning and establishment of a hybridoma producing a monoclonal antibody of interest. They are stored frozen, usually in liquid nitrogen vapour in a cell bank. These seed lots are reference samples of the hybridoma and therefore of its monoclonal antibody for future comparison of the characteristics of the hybridoma and its antibody as it is grown up *in vitro* or *in vivo* for actual production of antibody. On continued passage *in vitro* or *in vivo*, hybridomas may change the quality or quantity of antibody which they produce. Going back periodically to initiate new cultures from seed lot samples ensures that antibody of a consistent quality is produced. The establishment of a bank of seed lots of any one hybridoma is of particular importance if antibody is to be produced on a large scale and/or commercially.

Synthetic antigen. Isolation and characterisation of antigens, using among other technologies monoclonal antibodies, means that the molecular structure of the antigen or its epitope can now be identified. Such antigens, particularly those which are polypeptides, can now be produced synthetically and used as antigen for further immunisations to generate monoclonal antibodies.

Tissue culture. The culturing and growth of cells and tissues *in vitro*. The term is most widely used to refer to growth of cells, rather than organized tissue. Tissue culture is used for generating and culturing hybridomas producing monoclonal antibodies.

Titre. A measure of the strength of an antibody solution, or the concentration of antibody in serum. The titre is usually determined by a process of limiting dilution in which increasing dilutions of antibody are reacted with a fixed concentration of antigen. The greatest dilution still showing reaction is taken as the titre.

Transferrin. A plasma protein, important in iron transport. It will also bind indium, and radioindium can become attached to it in the circulation following breakdown of labelled antibodies.

Tumour-associated antigen. A broad term used to describe a material associated especially with malignant cells. The material may not be tumour-specific, and may only be expressed at higher levels on malignant rather than normal cells. The term *antigen* here is used really to show that the material is identified by reaction with an antibody, including monoclonal antibodies; it does not necessarily follow that the material is antigenic in the sense that the animal or patient with the tumour can produce an immune response against it. *Tumour marker* is really a better name for these materials, although that term is used most often to describe such material in the circulation where its detection by *in vitro* assays can be used in tumour diagnosis or monitoring.

Xenograft. Any graft of tissue between different species of animals. Xenografts of human tumours in mice, or occasionally rats, have been widely used to assess tumour localization and imaging properties of monoclonal antibodies. Depression of the animals' immune responses is necessary to allow the foreign tissue to grow, but now nude mice are commonly used.

Appendix: Antibody Look-Up Table

To those unfamiliar with monoclonal antibodies, their nomenclature may seem extremely confusing, with complex immunological terms and abbreviations mixed in with seemingly arbitrary code names. At the present time there is no agreed classification or international system of classification for monoclonal antibodies either as research materials or as clinical reagents. Hence, the definition of antibodies is often lacking, and the only means of obtaining information is by referral to original research publications. Monoclonal antibodies are generally referred to by code names which arise from a laboratory batch number assigned at the time of cell fusion, or according to designated product codes used by larger institutions or commercial organisations. Compilation of any form of comprehensive listing is a difficult and time-consuming task, and errors may occur due to a single antibody having been assigned different names or codes as a result of the material being exchanged between laboratories or released for commercial production. For example, the list includes an antibody designated 791T/36, this name being derived from the original immunogen (791T cells) and the cloning number. But this antibody is also known as NCRC-2 (being the second monoclonal antibody produced at Nottingham Cancer Research Campaign Laboratories). This antibody has been licenced to Xoma Corporation, California, USA, who have given it the name XMMCO-791.

Some antibodies are described in the literature simply by a number, and there is a possibility that quite different antibodies from different laboratories could have the same number! Even when names are different, there is still the possibility of confusion. Typical examples contained in the list below include an antibody M8 (against breast cancer associated antigen) and an antibody MAB8 (against lung cancer associated antigen). In some cases published data has been conflicting and the authors have had to use their discretion in the final listing. It is possible that different antibodies produced by different laboratories (but reacting with the same epitopes or an antigen) may be identical. The precise matching of these antibodies will only be possible after thorough characterisation studies have been carried out.

A list of the main antibodies that have shown potential for *in vivo* use is of value to new users of these materials and also provides a useful source of reference to the more experienced worker. The antibodies in this table are given in numerical and alphabetical order, stating the immunoglobulin isotype and the antigen where known. The list is not intended to be exhaustive, and to date not all the antibodies shown have been used *in vivo* clinically, although most have been evaluated in animal models. However, those listed are considered to be the prime candidates for clinical immunoscintigraphy in both benign and malignant diseases. A key reference is given so that the source and characteristics of the antibody may be obtained through published communications.

Antibody	Isotype	Antigen	Main application/potential	Key reference
103D2	IgG1	Breast (126kDa)	Ca breast	Khaw, J Nucl Med 25:592–603 (1984)
10E5	IgG2a	Platelet IIb/IIIa	Thrombus	Coller, J Clin Invest 72:325–338 (1983)
10F5.3	IgG2a	SCLC	SCLC	Stya, Proc Am Ass Cancer Res 26:292 (1985)
10F6.4	IgG2a	SCLC	SCLC	Stya, Proc Am Ass Cancer 26:292 (1985)
11.285.14	IgG1	CEA	Colorectal ca	Rowland, Cancer Immunol Immunother 21:183–187 (1986)
115	IgG1	CEA	Colorectal ca	Buchsbaum, Cancer Res 48:4324–4333 (1988)
149.53	IgG1	HMW MAA	Melanoma	Giacomini, Cancer Res 44:1281–1287 (1984)
16-88	IgM human monoclonal	Colon ca Ag	Colorectal ca	McCabe, Cancer Res 48:4348–4353 (1989)
161	IgG1	CEA/NCA	Colorectal ca	Pimm, Eur J Nucl Med 12:515–521 (1987)
17-1A	IgG2a	Undefined	Colorectal Ca	Mach, Cancer Res 43:5593–5600 (1983)
170H82		Pan adenocarcinoma	Adenocarcinoma	McEwan, Nucl Med Commun 11:206 (1990) Abstract
19-24	IgG1	Malignant histiocytoma	Sarcoma	Greager, Cancer Immunol Immunother 23:148–154 (1986)
19-24	IgG1	Sarcoma Ag	Soft tissue and bone sarcoma	Brown, J Natl Cancer Inst 15:637–644 (1985)
19-9	IgG1	200kDa Carbohydrate Ag	Ca pancreas, small bowel, ovary (mucinous)	Chatal, J Nucl Med 25:307–314 (1984)
198	IgG1	CEA/NCA	Colorectal ca	Pimm, Eur J Nucl Med 12:515–521 (1987)
1C12	IgG2a	CEA	Colorectal ca	Rogers, Eur J Cancer Clin Oncol 22:709–710 (1986)
1D4	IgG2a	Thyroglobulin	Thyroid ca	Shepherd, Eur J Nucl Med 10:291–295 (1985)
1H12		CEA	Colorectal ca	Rogers, Cancer Immunol Immunother 23:107–112 (1986)

(continued)

Antibody	Isotype	Antigen	Main application/potential	Key reference
202	IgG1	CEA	Colorectal ca	Buchsbaum, Eur J Nucl Med 10:398–402 (1985)
225.28S	IgG2a	HMW MAA (94kDa)	Melanoma	Burragi, J Nucl Med All Sci 28:283–295 (1984)
228	IgG2a	CEA/NCA	Colorectal ca	Pimm, Eur J Nucl Med 12:515–521 (1987)
250-30.6	IgG2b	Colon ca Ag	Colorectal ca	Zallbeng, J Natl Cancer Inst 71:801–808 (1983)
260F9	IgG1	Breast/ovary (55kDa)	Ca breast, ovary	Griffin, Cancer Immuno Immunother 29:43–50 (1989)
28A32	IgM human monoclonal	Colon Ca Ag	Colorectal Ca	McCabe, Cancer Res 48:4348–4353 (1989)
323/A3	IgG1	Breast (43kDa)	Ca breast	Khaw, Eur J Nucl Med 14:362–366 (1988)
38S1	IgG1	Colon LS174T Ag	Ca colon	Hedin, Int J Cancer 30:547–552 (1982)
3E1-2	IgM	Breast ca	Ca breast	Thompson, Lancet ii 1245–1247 (1984)
3F8	IgG3	GD2 ganglioside	Neuroblastoma	Miraldi, Radiology 161:431–418 (1986)
425	IgG2a	EGF receptor	EGF producing tumours	Takahashi, Cancer Res 47:3847–3850 (1987)
431/31(TUMAK)	IgG1	CEA	Ca ovary	Duewell, Cancer Immunol Immunother 23:101–106 (1986)
454A12	IgG1	Breast/ovary ca Ag	Ca breast, ovary	Marks, Cancer Res 50:288–292 (1990)
465.12S	IgG2a	Cytoplasmic MAA	Melanoma	Giacomini, Cancer Res 44:1281–1287 (1984)
48.7	IgG1	HMW MAA	Melanoma	Larson, Cancer Invest 2:363–381 (1984)
4F7.4	IgG2a	SCLC	SCLC	Stya, Proc Am Ass Cancer Res 26:292 (1985)
50H.19	IgG1	Platelet IIb/IIIa	Thrombus	Oster, Nucl Med Commun 9:843–847 (1988)
543F8	IgM	SCLC	SCLC	Cuttita, Proc Natl Acad Sci (USA) 78:4591–4895 (1981)
59D8	IgG1	Fibrin II	Thrombus	Knight, LC Nucl Med Commun 9:823–829 (1988)

Antibody	Ig class	Antigen	Target	Reference
5G11	IgG2a	Thrombospondin	Thrombus	Legrand, Eur J Biochem 171:393–399 (1988)
5G6.4	IgG2a	Epithelial OvCa	Ca ovary	Whal, J Nucl Med 30:60–65 (1989)
600D11	IgM	SCLC/NSCLC	Ca lung (mixed)	Rossen, Cancer Res 44:2052–2059 (1984)
604A6	IgM	SCLC (31kDa)	SCLC	Cuttita, Proc Natl Acad Sci (USA) 78:4591–4895 (1981)
64C5	IgM	Fibrin II	Thrombus	Hui, Thromb Haemost 54:524–527 (1985)
763.74T	IgG1	HMW MAA	Melanoma	Giacomini, Cancer Res 44:1281–1287 (1984)
791T/36	IgG2b	72kDa Gp	Ca, colon, ovary, breast, lung, bone tumours	Armitage, Br J Surg 71:407–412 (1984)
7E3	IgG	Platelet IIb/IIIa	Thrombus	Coller, J Clin Invest 72:325–338 (1983)
8.2.	IgG1	p97Da MAA	Melanoma	Larson, J Nucl Med 24:123–129 (1983)
81C6	IgG2b	Neuroectodermal tissue	Neuroblastoma	Zalutsky, Cancer Res 49:2807–2813 (1989)
9.2.2.	IgM	SqCLC	SqCLC	Brenner, Cancer Res 42:3187–3192 (1982)
9.2.27	IgG2a	MAA (250kDa)	Melanoma	Eary, J Nucl Med 30:25–32 (1989)
96.5	IgG2a	p97Da MAA	Melanoma	Larson, J Nucl Med 24:123–129 (1983)
A3	IgG1	PLAP (57kDa)	Ca ovary	Jemmerson & Stigbrand, FEBS lett 173–357–359 (1984)
A6H	IgG1	Renal cell ca Ag	Renal cell ca	Vesellia, Nat Cancer Inst Monogram 3:159–167 (1987)
AF01	IgG2	AFP	Ca ovary, testes, hepatoma	Demangeat, Eur J Nucl Med 14:612–620 (1988)
AF04	IgG1	AFP	Ca ovary, testes, hepatoma	Demangeat, Eur J Nucl Med 14:612–620 (1988)
AF08	IgG1	AFP	Hepatoma	Manil, J Immunol Methods 90:25–37 (1986)
Anti-B1	IgG2a	CD20 of B cells	Lymphoma	Buchsbaum, Cancer Res 48:2475–2482 (1988)
Anti-HCG	IgG1	β-HCG	HCG producing tumours	Behring, Personal communication, R P Baum University Hospital Frankfurt FRG
Anti-HT6	IgG1	Thyroglobulin	Ca thyroid	Behring, Personal communication, R P Baum University Hospital Frankfurt FRG

(continued)

Antibody	Isotype	Antigen	Main application/potential	Key reference
Anti-J5	IgG2a	CD10 lymphoma Ag	Lymphoma	Buchsbaum, Cancer Res 48:2475–2482 (1988)
ASB7		CEA	Colorectal ca	Pedley, Brit J Cancer 60:549–554 (1989)
AUA1	IgG1	Epithelial proliferating Ag	Ca ovary	Epenetos, Br J Cancer 46:1–8 (1982)
B6.2	IgG	Breast	Ca breast	Colcher, Cancer Res 43:736–742 (1983)
B72.3	IgG1	TAG-72	Ca colon, ovary	Estaban, Int J Cancer 39:50–59 (1987)
BA-1	IgM	Leukaemia Ag	Leukaemia	Buchsbaum, Eur J Nucl Med 10:398–402 (1985)
BW111	IgG1	Pan-T-lymphocyte	Lymphoma	Behring, Personal communication, R P Baum University Hospital Frankfurt FRG
BW250/183 Granulozyt	IgG1	NCA-(95kDa)/CEA	Granulocyte labelling	Lind, J Nucl Med 31:417–423 (1990)
BW431/26	IgG1	CEA (180kDa)	Colorectal ca	Baum, Nucl Med Commun 10:345–352 (1989)
BW431/31	IgG1	CEA (180kDa)	Colorectal ca	Behring, Personal communication, R P Baum University Hospital Frankfurt FRG
BW436/20	IgG1	Monocytes	Chronic inflammation	Behring, Personal communication, R P Baum University Hospital Frankfurt FRG
BW494/32	IgGl	Mucin (>200kDa)	Ca pancreas, ovary	Bosslet, Cancer Immunol Immunother 23:185–191 (1986)
BW575/100	IgG1	Lung	Ca lung	Behring, Personal communication, R P Baum University Hospital Frankfurt FRG
BW575/9	IgGl	90kDa Gp	Neuroblastoma	Baum, Eur J Nucl Med 15:C3 (1989) Abstract
BW625	IgG3	Ganglioside GD2	Glioma	Bosslet, Cancer Immuno Immunother 29:171–178 (1989)
BW704	IgG3	Ganglioside GD2	Glioma	Bosslet, Cancer Immuno Immunother 29:171–178 (1989)
C24/1/39	IgG1	CEA	Colorectal ca	Andrew, Eur J Nucl Med 12:168–175 (1986)

Clone	Ig class	Antigen	Target	Reference
C4	IgG2b	PLAP (57kDa)	Ca ovary	Jemmerson & Stigbrand, FEBS lett 173:357–359 (1984)
C42032		Undefined	GI and mammary tumours	Herlyn, Cancer Res 43:2731–2735 (1983)
C46	IgG2a	CEA	Colorectal ca	Armitage, Br J Surg 73:965–969 (1988)
C5H	IgG1	Renal cell ca Ag	Renal cell ca	Vesellia, Nat Cancer Inst Monogram 3:159–167 (1987)
CD37	IGg2a	Pan-B cells (40/45kDa)	Lymphoma	Loutfi, Nucl Med Commun 9:787–796 (1988)
CEI-326	IgG1	CEA	Colorectal ca	Hagan, J Nucl Med 26:1418–1423 (1985)
CHA255	IgG1	In 3+ chelate	Chelate specific	Goodwin, Nucl Med Commun 7:569–580 (1986)
CHB235	IgG1	In 3+ chelate	Chelate specific	Goodwin, Nucl Med Commun 7:569–580 (1986)
CO29.11	IgG1	Lewis A antigen	Colorectal Ca	Mung, L Nucl Med 27:1739–1745 (1986)
CT03	IyG1	26-32 Calcitonin	Medullary thyroid Ca	Manil, Cancer Res 49:5480–5485 (1989)
CT06	IgG1	11-17 Calcitonin	Medullary thyroid Ca	Manil, Cancer Res 49:5480–5485 (1989)
CT14	IgG1	C-myc oncogene	Ca lung	Chan, Br J Cancer 54:761–769 (1986)
D2OL		PLAP	Ca ovary	Epenetos, Br J Cancer 49:11–15 (1984)
D612	IgG2a	1000kDa Gp	Colorectal ca	Mottolese, Br J Cancer 61:626–630 (1990)
DD-3B6-22		Fibrin II	Thrombus	Knight, LC Nucl Med Commun 9:823–829 (1988)
DU-PAN-1	IgG2	HMW Gp(pancreatic)	Ca pancreas	Metzgar, Cancer Res 42:601–608 (1982)
DU-PAN-2	IgM	Pancreatic duct	Ca pancreas	Metzgar, Cancer Res 42:601–608 (1982)
DU-PAN-3	IgG2	70kDa Gp	Ca pancreas	Metzgar, Cancer Res 42:601–608 (1982)
DU-PAN-4	IgG1		Ca pancreas	Metzgar, Cancer Res 42:601–608 (1982)
DU-PAN-5	IgG1	110kDa Gp	Ca pancreas	Metzgar, Cancer Res 42:601–608 (1982)

(continued)

Antibody	Isotype	Antigen	Main application/potential	Key reference
E5	IgG2a	PLAP (57kDa)	Ca ovary	Jemmerson & Stigbrand, FEBS lett 173:357–359 (1984)
F6	IgG2a	PLAP (57kDa)	Ca ovary	Jemmerson & Stigbrand, FEBS lett 173:357–359 (1984)
FB12	IgG1	HCG	Ca ovary	Demangeat, Eur J Nucl Med 14:612–620 (1988)
FO23C5	IgG1	CEA	Colorectal ca	Siccardi, Cancer Res 49:3095–3103 (1989)
GA73-3	IgG2a	Adenoca (29, 30 and 37kDa)	Colorectal Ca	Munz, L Nucl Med 27:1739–1745 (1986)
Granuloszint MABgc(MABA47)	IgGl	NCA (95kDaGp)/CEA	Granulocyte labelling	Seybold, Nucl Med Commun 9:745–752 (1988)
H17E2	IgG1	PLAP	Ca ovary	Epenetos, Br J Radiology 59:117–125 (1986)
H317	IgG1	PLAP	Ca ovary	Epenetos, Br J Radiology 59:117–125 (1986)
H7	IgG2a	PLAP (57kDa)	Ca ovary	Jemmerson & Stigbrand, FEBS lett 173:357–359 (1984)
HMFG1	IgG1	GpAg	Ca ovary	Epenetos, Lancet 2:999–1005 (1982)
HMFG2	IgG1	GpAg	Ca ovary	Granowska, Nucl Med Communs: 485–499 (1984)
KCO1	IgG1	Katacalcin (PDN21)	Medullary thyroid Ca	Manil, Cancer Res 49:5480–5484 (1989)
KS1/4 LS20207 LON/HT13	IgG2a	40kDaGp Adenoca Ag Teratoma Ag	Ca lung ovary bowel Adenocarcinoma (mixed) Teratoma	Vakey, Cancer Res 44:681–685 (1984) Brown, Radiology 173:701–705 (1989) Moshakis, Brit J Cancer 44:663–669 (1981)
LYM-1	IgG2a	Burkitts lymphoma	Lymphoma	Adams, Cancer Res 49:1707–1711 (1989)
M8	IgGl	EMA	Ca breast	Rainsbury, Br J Surg 71:805–812 (1984)
MA5	IgG1	EMA	Ca breast	Major, Eur J Nucl Med 15:655–660 (1989)
Mab19-24	IgG1	Osteosarcoma Ag	Osteosarcoma	Greayer, J Clin Immunol Immunother 23:148–154 (1986)

Antibody	Ig	Antigen	Target	Reference
Mab35	IgG1	CEA	Colorectal ca	Delaloye, J Clin Invest 71:301–311 (1986)
Mab8	IgG3	Lung ca	Lung ca	Endo, Cancer Res 47:5427–5432 (1987)
MOV16	IgG1	OvCa (50kDaGp)	Ca ovary	Miotti, Int J Cancer 39:297–303 (1987)
MOV18	IgG1	40kDaGp	Ca ovary	Burraggi, Eur J Nucl Med 14:C5 (1988) Abstract
MOV19	IgG2a	OvCa (40kDaGp)	Ca ovary	Miotti, Int J Cancer 39:297–303 (1987)
NDGO2	IgG2a	PLAP	Ca ovary	Jackson, Eur J Nucl Med 11:22–28 (1985)
NP-2		CEA	Colorectal ca	Fand, Cancer Res 47:2177–2183 (1987)
OC-125	IgG1	CA-125(75kDa)	Ca ovary (serous)	Chatal, J Nucl Med 26:149–190 (1987)
OST15	IgG2a	Osteosarcoma Ag	Osteosarcoma	Koizumi, Cancer Res 49:1752–1757 (1989)
OST6	IgG1	Osteosarcoma Ag	Osteosarcoma	Koizumi, Cancer Res 49:1752–1757 (1989)
OST7	IgG	Osteosarcoma Ag	Bone tumours	Sakahara, J Nucl Med 28:342–348 (1987)
OVTL-3	IgG	OvCa	Ca ovary	Massuger, Eur J Nucl Med 15:C1 (1989) Abstract
P256	IgG1	Platelet IIb/IIIa	Thrombus	Peters, Br M J 29:1525–1527 (1986)
PA7276	IGg2a	Prostate acid phosphotase	Ca prostate	Babaian, J Urol 137:439–443 (1987)
Po66	IgG1	LSqCC	LSqCC	Dazord, Cancer Immunol Immunother 24:263–268 (1987)
PRIA3	IgG1	Epithelial cell surface antigen	Colorectal ca	Granowska, Eur J Nucl Med 15:C5 (1989) Abstract
R11D10/Myoscint	IgG2a	Myosin	Myocardial infarct, rhabdomyosarcoma	Khaw, Science 209:295–297 (1980)
RCC-1	IgG2a	Breast ca Ag	Ca breast	Tjardra, Cancer Res 49:1600–1608 (1989)
S12	IgG	Platelet IIb/IIIa	Thrombus	McEver & Martin, J Biol Chem 259:9799–9804 (1984)
SCCL-114	IgM	SCLC	SCLC	Ball, J Natl Cancer Inst 72:593–598 (1984)

(continued)

Antibody	Isotype	Antigen	Main application/potential	Key reference
SCCL-124	IgM	SCLC	SCLC	Ball, J Natl Cancer Inst 72:593–598 (1984)
SCCL-175	IgM	SCLC	SCLC	Memoli, Cancer Res 48:7319–7322 (1988)
SCCL-41	IgM	SCLC	SCLC	Ball, J Natl Cancer Inst 72:593–598 (1984)
SM3	IgG1	Stripped mucin	Colorectal ca	Burchell, Cancer Res 47:5476–5482 (1987)
SWA11	IgG2a	SCLC	SCLC	Smith, Br J Cancer 59:174–178 (1989)
SWA20	IgG2a	SCLC	SCLC	Smith, Br J Cancer 59:174–178 (1989)
SWA21	IgG	SCLC	SCLC	Smith, Br J Cancer 59:174–178 (1989)
SWA22	IgG	SCLC	SCLC	Smith, Br J Cancer 59:174–178 (1989)
T101	IGg2a	T cell-T65	T cell lymophoma	Carrasquillo, J Nucl Med 28:281–287 (1987)
T2G1s	IGg1	Fibrin II	Thrombus	Knight, LC Nucl Med Commun 9:823–829 (1988)
T84.12	IgG2a	CEA	Colorectal ca	Beatty, Cancer Res 49:1587–1584 (1989)
T84.66	IgG1	CEA	Colorectal ca	Beatty, Cancer Res 49:1587–1584 (1989)
TA99	IgG2a	MAA Gp	Melanoma	Welt, Proc Nat Acad Sci 84:4200–4204 (1981)
TF5S-4	IgG1	SCLC	SCLC	Watnabe, Cancer Res 47:826–829 (1987)
TFS-1	IgG2a	SCLC/NSCLC (42kDa)	Ca lung (mixed)	Okabe, Cancer Res 44:5273–5278 (1984)
TFS-2	IgG2b	SCLC/NSCLC (39kDa)	Ca lung (mixed)	Okabe, Cancer Res 44:5273–5278 (1984)
TFS-3	IgG1	SCLC/NSCLC (110kDa)	Ca lung (mixed)	Okabe, Cancer Res 44:5273–5278 (1984)
TFS-4	IgG1	SCLC/NSCLC (124kDa)	Ca lung (mixed)	Okabe, Cancer Res 44:5273–5278 (1984)
Tg03(211/A5)	IgG2a	Thyroglobulin	Ca thyroid	Bellet, J Clin Endocrinal Metab 56:530–533 (1983)

Name	Isotype	Antigen	Disease	Reference
TP-1	IgG2a	Osteosarcoma Ag	Osteosarcoma	Bruland, Brit J Cancer 56:21–25 (1987)
TP-3	IgG2b	Osteosarcoma Ag	Osteosarcoma	Bruland, Brit J Cancer 56:21–25 (1987)
UCHT2	IgG1	Pan-T cells (67kDa)	Lymphoma	Loutfi, Nucl Med Commun 9:787–796 (1988)
UJI3A	IgG1	Neuroectodermal tissue	Neural tumours	Goldman, J Paediatrics 105:252–256 (1984)
VII-23		CEA	Colorectal ca	Berche, Br Med J 285:1447–1451 (1982)
W14A	IgG1	HCG	HCG producing tumours	Searle, Cancer Immunoc Immunother 21:205–208 (1986)
WML-34		Mycobacterium TB	TB	Hazra, Nucl Med Commun 8:139–142 (1987)
WTB-72		Mycobacterium TB	TB	Hazra, Nucl Med Commun 8:139–142 (1987)
XMMME-001	IgG2a	HMW MAA	Melanoma	Elliot, Br J Cancer 59:600–604 (1989)
YBM-209	IgM human monoclonal	Ca breast	Ca breast	Ryan, Radiology 167:71–75 (1988)
YBY-088	IgM human monoclonal	Ca breast	Ca breast	Ryan, Radiology, 167:71–75 (1988)
YPC/12.1	IgG2a rat monoclonal	Colon/breast	Ca colon/breast	Smedley, Br J Cancer 47:253–259 (1983)
YPC2/38.8	Rat monoclonal	Colon & liver ca Ag	Colorectal ca	Markham, J Hepatology 2:25–31 (1986)
ZCE-025(MAB35)	IGg1	CEA (180kDa)	Colorectal ca	Abel-Nabi, Radiology 164:617–621 (1987)
ZCE/CHA	IgG1	CEA/bleomycin bispecific monoclonal	Colorectal ca	Stickney, Antibody Immunoconjugates & Radiopharmaceuticals 2:1–13 (1989)
ZME-018	IgG2a	240kDa Gp MAA	Melanoma	Murray, J Nucl Med 28:25–33 (1987)

Index